THE THRIFTY GIRL'S GUIDE TO GLAMOUR

LIVING THE

Beautiful Life

ON LITTLE OR

NO MONEY

Susie Galvez

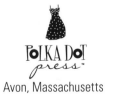

POLKA DOT
press

Avon, Massachusetts

Published by
Polk Dot Press, and imprint of Adams Media,
an F+W Publications Company
57 Littlefield Street
Avon, MA 02322
www.adamsmedia.com

ISBN 10: 1-59337-622-7
ISBN 13: 978-1-59337-622-2

Printed in the United States of America.

J   I   H   G   F   E   D   C   B   A

Library of Congress Cataloging-in-Publication Data
Galvez, Susie.
The thrifty girl's guide to glamour / Susie Galvez.
p.   cm.
ISBN-13: 978-1-59337-622-2
ISBN-10: 1-59337-622-7
1. Beauty, Personal. 2. Cosmetics. I. Title.

RA778.G328 2006
646.7'042--dc22

2006019983

This publication is designed to provide accurate and authoritative information with regard to the subject matter covered. It is sold with the understanding that the publisher is not engaged in rendering legal, accounting, or other professional advice. If legal advice or other expert assistance is required, the services of a competent professional person should be sought.
—From a *Declaration of Principles* jointly adopted by a Committee of the American Bar Association and a Committee of Publishers and Associations

Many of the designations used by manufacturers and sellers to distinguish their product are claimed as trademarks. Where those designations appear in this book and Adams Media was aware of a trademark claim, the designations have been printed with initial capital letters.

This book is available at quantity discounts for bulk purchases.
For information, please call 1-800-872-5627.

Special Appreciation

"One can never pay in gratitude;
one can only pay 'in kind' somewhere else in life."

—ANNE MORROW LINDBERGH

This book could not have been completed without the unwavering support and love from my very special friends. Thank you to:

Paula Munier, who believed in me.

Meredith O'Hayre, who believed in my words.

Anne Szamboti, Judith Ann Graham, Melissa Laine, Bonnie Risley, Lisa Krizan, and **Susie Hayman,** who have allowed me to test on them every beauty concoction I could come up with.

Veronica Brockwell, for sharing my vision.

Richard Nicolo, for understanding my passion—and bottling it.

Amy Nicolo, for the know-how to get it done.

Kimberly Frey, who loves "all things cosmetic" as much as I do.

And lastley, but always first with me, thank you, **Tino Galvez**—you are truly the wind beneath my wings. XOXO.

CONTENTS

Introduction

" Glamour is something no woman can be born with. It is not a gift at all. It is more of a concoction than anything else. **"**

—LORETTA YOUNG

I guess you could say that I was born to blush, or least to apply it. My love for beauty began while sitting at my mother's dressing table at the age of five. All of the beautiful bottles of potions and lotions, which, if I close my eyes, I can still see, continue to fascinate me even today.

My own glamorous life started a little later—at my seventh-grade grammar school graduation. My mother surprised me with my graduation outfit: the most beautiful pink (just like the color of this book cover) shirtwaist dress, with a full skirt that would twirl when I spun around; pink patent leather pumps with kitten heels, sheer hosiery (the first time ever I was allowed to shave my legs!), and the prettiest shade of Ballerina Pink lipstick that you have ever seen (lipstick, also a first).

As I walked across the gymnasium floor to receive my diploma from Mr. Otts, the principal, it felt like I was on the red carpet and accepting the most glamorous girl in the world award. I will never forget that moment.

Glamour is like that. It is the feeling that you get when you know that you look beautiful from head to toe and feel absolutely wonderful in your own skin. *The Thrifty Girl's Guide to Glamour*'s goal is to help you create your own glamour moments—on a daily basis.

My dream is for you to read a tip or two and say, "You know what? I can do that." Or, even better for me is to have you say, "You know what? I used to do that—I want to do that again!" Please use this book as your personal glamour resource guide. Enjoy your beauty moments and, most of all, enjoy yourself!

And as I always close my beauty speech presentations: "Always remember, a little powder and a little paint—helps you look like what you ain't!"

Surround yourself with beauty!

PART 1

THE
THRIFTY
GIRL'S
GUIDE TO
GLAMOROUS
HAIR

This section of *The Thrifty Girl's Guide to Glamour* is devoted to achieving a glamorous 'do. From color, cut, and style to the most flattering styles for your face, this section covers it all.

Chapter One

In Living Color

If you want a head of hair that stands out in a crowd, look no further than color. Hair color holds the power to make almost anyone glamorous. Many celebrities, marketing mavens, and advertising gurus are firm believers in the idea that if you change your hair color, you instantly transform your life. It is estimated that three-quarters of women use hair color as a way to boost their confidence both in their working and personal lives. Want a little lift? Add a little color.

GUINEA PIGS WANTED

While salon coloring sessions can be very pricey (anywhere from $60 to over $300), you can still luck upon a bargain or two. Here are a couple different ways you can score a new color for little or no money at all!

Workshops in Beauty Salons

The world of coloring is always changing, so true beauty professionals must keep up by attending color classes. In most cases, different professional hair color companies visit salons to show the staff the latest in colors and techniques. If you are willing to be a test model, a new hue is awaiting you for free. Simply call around to the salons and spas near you and tell them you are more than happy to be a model for upcoming classes. Who knows, you might even score a new haircut as well!

Beauty Schools

Beauty schools are also excellent ways to discover the world of color without a high price tag. After students graduate from mannequins to real heads, they are always in search of live ones to show off what they have learned. While they are indeed students, you have a safety net, as the teacher is never far away. For the price of a latte and scone, you can have a new lease on life with a wonderful new color.

COLORING AT HOME

If you are thinking, "I just would rather do it myself," know that coloring the hair at home can be a bit tricky—but very doable. While the process could take as little as an hour to go from box to blow-dry, coloring projects undertaken in haste could result in months of growing-out regrets. Although complicated coloring projects—such as weaving different colors—are best left to the professionals, with some careful planning, a list of *realistic* expectations, and a little patience, new shades of beautiful blonde, razzle-dazzle red, and bombshell brown are just an afternoon away!

GO AHEAD—WIG OUT!

Before going color-crazy, why not first try on a wig to see if the color suits you? Scarlet Red or Raven Black tresses may be what you have pictured in your mind's eye, but they create quite a different look when you see yourself up close and personal. Trying on wigs offers a fun, free, and fail-safe way to explore the depths of color before taking the plunge. Try on several and take some photos. Who knows, you may find out that you look fabulous in lots of shades!

Home hair coloring has become far more sophisticated than what was found on the store shelves even just a few years ago—but *care* is still the word for the wise, so as to not end up with "supermarket hair." Supermarket hair is distinctly noticeable hair that is too bright, too dark, or a completely solid color with no nuances of definition. In fact, it looks about as flat as the box it came in!

Thrifty Girls know that a good value must be matched with good knowledge. Here is the lowdown on the highlights:

TEMPORARY: Lasts through one or two shampoos. The colorants coat the outside of the cuticle and do not usually contain peroxide or ammonia. Temporary colors will not remove any natural color from the hair but will deepen, brighten, or enhance what already exists. My favorite types of temporary color are:

- John Frieda Luminous Color Glaze
- L'Oreal Colour Pulse

SEMI-PERMANENT: Lasts through four to six shampoos. Like temporary color, these products color the outside of the hair shaft and down to the next layer. These products are also typically free of peroxide or ammonia. Because the color covers one layer of the hair, it may last longer on fine hair. My favorite semi-permanent dye?

- Clairol Loving Care

DEMI-PERMANENT: Lingers for up to twenty shampoos. This hair coloring formula deposits color between the hair cuticle and cortex and may contain some peroxide or ammonia to remove some natural color. Looking for a demi-permanent fix? Try:

- Clairol Natural Instinct

PERMANENT: The hair cuticle is opened and the color is deposited onto the cortex. These color formulas contain peroxide and ammonia. The color lasts until it grows out, is cut off, or is recolored. Ready for a permanent overhaul? Try:

- Preference L'Oreal
- Clairol Hydrience
- Revlon High Dimension
- Garnier Nutrisse

HIGHLIGHTS: These color formulas lift pigments from the hair cortex and contain peroxide, bleach, or ammonia. Want to try out some highlights? Why not try:

- L'Oreal Couleur Experte
- L'Oreal Couleur Strands Quick Shimmer
- L'Oreal Excellence

DOUBLE PROCESS COLOR: These products open the cuticle so the hair can be lightened four to six levels (or shades) with peroxide, ammonia, or bleach. New color is then deposited via a toner into the hair cortex through the cuticle. If you're interested in trying a double process color, my favorites are:

- Clairol Xtreme FX
- L'Oreal Feria
- Garnier 100% Color

While temporary, semi- and demi-permanent hues are generally considered safe for most tresses, there are always exceptions to every hair rule. In some situations, washout tones may become permanent if applied to strands that are porous or damaged from previous bleaching or chemical treatments.

THRIFTY TIP

If you are new to the home hair coloring game, you might want to try temporary, semi- or demi-permanent color. Then if, knock on wood, you make a mistake, the evidence can be washed down the drain in just a few shampoos. Once you get the handle on hair color, you can step up to the permanent ones.

After you have decided on the right color formula, evaluate the best shade for your age, skin tone, facial features, and lifestyle. Here are some tips to help you cast the dye:

- Remember that hair color can lift and lighten, match existing colors and brighten, or provide depth through darker, richer hues.
- Choose colors that are soft, natural, and classy. Consider shades that will slightly lighten, brighten, or deepen your current hair tone.
- Shades that are no more than two shades lighter or darker than your current hair color will blend the best. The rule of two—only two shades up or down—will help avoid a sharp demarcation color line when your roots emerge.
- Act your age. Colors that are marketed to much younger consumers are not designed to cover gray and will be too bright for the over-thirties crowd's skin tone and eye coloring.
- Keep away from the dark side. Very dark shades will intensify the signs of aging. To look younger, go one to two shades lighter.
- Consider purchasing an extra hair color kit, especially if your hair is long and/or thick. You might have to use two kits to get the coverage complete. Save the receipt, and you can return it if you don't need it. It sure beats driving back to the store with a towel on your head!

Once you have selected the hair color product and shade perfect for you—take a few color cues:

- Check the hair color box expiration date to ensure that the product is still viable.
- When you arrive home, take out everything in the box and read the instructions twice.
- Don't go by the model on the box cover. Instead use the color chart included in the instructions to determine what shade you can realistically expect to end up with.
- If you have not used color on your hair before, it is best to do a patch test at least 48 hours before you color to avoid any unexpected allergic reactions.
- Dress for the occasion. Put on an old shirt and put a towel over your shoulders.
- Always color on clean, dry hair. Styling products can leave residue that could affect the color.
- If you use styling products routinely, consider using a clarifying shampoo at least one week before using home hair color. This will help remove any excess product layered onto the cuticle.
- Always wear gloves. If you don't like the ones in the box, purchase a pair of coloring gloves. They can be found at beauty supply stores.
- If you color at home on a regular basis, a hair coloring brush is a good investment.
- Apply a thin layer of Vaseline around your hairline and the tips of your ears to prevent staining.
- To ensure uniform coverage, begin applying color at the back of the head and work forward.
- Ask a friend over. If this is your first time coloring your hair, consider asking a friend over to help you to make sure you don't miss a spot. Plus, it is fun for a glamour girl to share in the beauty makeover.

- When the color has finished developing, shampoo and rinse out the remaining product as described in the instructions. Hair color is designed to stop processing at a set point—leaving it in your hair longer will not alter when the processing is finished.
- Dispose of any leftover color as soon as you are finished. Unused amounts cannot be used at a later date. And do not under any circumstances color your eyebrows with hair color. Doing so is a serious blindness risk!
- In the event of a coloring mishap, call the hotline telephone number from the back of the box *before* doing anything else.

Maintaining Your Glamorous— and Thrifty—New 'Do

You have now achieved your totally glamorous color. After spending a little mirror time enjoying the new you, follow some tips for keeping the 'do darling:

- Wait forty-eight hours before washing your hair after you color. The hair needs time to settle.
- Shampoo with warm, not hot, water. Water that is too hot will cause the color to fade more quickly.
- Hair products designed for color-treated hair are best and will keep the color longer. FYI: Volume-building shampoos can cause the color to fade faster, as the volumizers open up the hair cuticle, which allows color to be washed out.
- Linger longer. Shampooing the hair less will pay off in color that is longer lasting and better conditioned. See if you can stretch it a day longer than you normally would.
- Keep the heat from the styling appliances on a lower setting. The higher the setting, the more damaging it is to treated hair.

- Wearing a hat when out in the sun or a cap while swimming will keep the sun, surf, sand, and pool chemicals from affecting the color.
- Treat colored hair with tender loving care. Use the best products you afford.
- A deep conditioning treatment on a regular basis will keep the hair looking and feeling great.
- Wait at least one month before attempting any other chemical processes, such as perming or straightening, as these products will change the color.

If your budget will allow it, try to schedule a color session with a professional every fourth or fifth coloring to keep your color looking rich and glamorous. The professional will be able to make sure that your hair color is uniform and not straying toward the brassy or ashy tones.

Benefits of Doing Your Own 'Do

Home hair coloring has many advantages. First of course, there is the price: under $10. Plus, often the home color companies will offer coupons in magazines, in the newspaper, and even at the store itself, allowing for an even bigger bang for your buck.

LIVING THE HIGH(LIGHT) LIFE

Switching from all-over color to highlights allows you to save more time and money. The average all-over color treatment is done every three to four weeks. Highlights grow out subtly. You can go as long as twelve weeks between coloring sessions.

Coloring your hair at home also allows you to multitask if you want to. While your hair is processing, you can read your mail, chat with a friend on the phone, give yourself a pedicure, or, if you are in the mood, you could even organize your closet—then again, maybe not.

Chapter Two

Flattery Will Get You Everywhere

" Flattery seldom falls flat. "

—UNKNOWN

W e've all been there. You go to your favorite salon, sit in front of the hairstylist you've come to trust your tresses to, and once the smock is removed and the last hair blown dry, you look up to realize that you've just woken up in a hair nightmare. The cut is not what you asked for, or maybe you asked for the wrong thing. To be a true thrifty girl, you have to prevent expensive mistakes before they happen. This chapter will help you avoid the most common hair mishap: getting a haircut that does not flatter your face.

One of the most basic questions when selecting the most flattering hairstyle is: What is your facial shape? Depending on which beauty expert you ask, the common shapes are oval, round, heart, square, and rectangle. And if that's not confusing enough, two new shapes have been added to the facial shape list. They are the pear (or reversed heart shape) and the triangle (or diamond shape). Let's see where you fall in the spectrum.

FACIAL SHAPE FLATTERY

To discover your own facial shape, you can take an instant photo of your face with your hair pulled back, or with a headband on. Have someone take your photo while you look straight into the camera. Instruct them to focus on photographing just your head and neck. Look at the photo and trace the outline of your face with a colorful marker, thus revealing your facial shape.

PARTING WAYS

Did you know that your hair part sends out signals about your personality? Who would have thought it? A part on the right side says that you are a gentle and caring person. A part on the extreme left part of the head makes you look more assertive and intelligent. A center part indicates that you are trustworthy. I wonder what the popular zigzag part is saying!

If you don't have an instant camera handy, or a friend to capture the moment, a quick way to determine your facial shape is to try the mirror trick. With your hair pulled away from your face, stand in front of your mirror. Take a lipstick (one that you never liked anyway) or a dry erase marker and at arm's length, draw lightly around the outline of your face on the mirror. Study the facial outline and see which of the following shapes best suits your face and which hairstyles will keep the flattery coming.

Oval

Oval faces appear only slightly narrower at the jaw line than at the temples, with a gently rounded hairline.

Flattering

Almost any length or style works well for this classic shape. The lucky oval facial shape can wear more styles than any other face shape can. You can wear your hair styled short, medium, or long. Hair pulled away from the face shows off the symmetrical oval. Try a classic long style with a center or side part and hair cascading to the shoulders. This shape looks great with layers designed to show off other facial features such as great cheekbones, beautiful eyes, exquisite chin, or luscious lips.

Avoid

Styles that add too much height near the crown take away from your "perfect" oval features. Covering your face with heavy bangs, or hair-forward-directed styles, is not your best look.

FAMOUS FACES: OVAL SHAPE

Some famous oval facial shapes are Jennifer Aniston, Cameron Diaz, Mariah Carey, Cindy Crawford, Jewel, Heather Locklear, Sharon Stone, Uma Thurman, Tyra Banks, Courtney Cox Arquette, and Elle MacPherson.

Round

Round faces consist of a full-looking face with a round chin and hairline. The widest point is at the cheeks and ears.

Flattering

Focus on chiseling the width of the face by adding side-swept bangs, and longer layers, shaggy, or tapered styles that caress the cheeks. This facial shape can carry hairstyles with fullness and height at the crown very well. Off-center parts, short hairstyles with a swept-back direction, or hairstyles that are longer than chin length also work very well.

By layering the top to achieve fullness and keeping the rest of the cut relatively close to the face, the round facial shape will appear longer and narrower.

Avoid

Chin-length hair with a rounded line that bends into the facial shape will make the face appear wider and fuller. Because the widest part of the face is at the cheeks and ears, avoiding having the fullness of the cut here will be more flattering.

Center parts, short-short crops, straight "chopped" bangs, or do's with fullness at the side of the ears are not your most complimenting look.

FAMOUS FACES: ROUND SHAPE

Round facial shapes on the red carpet include Ingrid Bergman, Drew Barrymore, Kate Winslet, Charlotte Church, Catherine Zeta Jones, and Christina Ricci.

Heart

Heart faces are wide at the temples and hairline, narrowing to a small delicate chin.

Flattering

Concentrate on styles that add width from the jawline downward to balance a pointy or prominent chin. A chin-length bob is great on your facial shape! This creates a balanced look by giving fullness where you need it. Since the heart-shaped face is widest across the forehead and temple area, consider experimenting with side-swept fringes or deep side parts that will visually break up the width.

You can wear shorter hairstyles; however, if you are a dramatic heart-shaped face, you need to leave weight in the back nape area. This will achieve more balance between your dramatic cheekbones and more narrowing chin.

Avoid

Short, full styles with tapered necklines will emphasize the upper face and make you look top heavy. Too much height at the crown will give the appearance of a longer and narrower chin.

Just remember if you have a dramatic heart-shaped face, you have great cheekbones to emphasize. Don't miss the beauty boat by getting a style that is too top-heavy.

FAMOUS FACES: HEART SHAPE

Heart facial shapes on the big screen include Michelle Pfeiffer, Ashley Judd, Jennifer Love Hewitt, Naomi Campbell, Juliette Binoche, Lisa Kudrow, and Lucy Lawless.

Square

Square-shaped faces have a strong, square jawline and usually an equally square hairline.

Take the edge off the sharp edges and angles of the face with soft, muted layers and rounded hairstyles. Try a side-swept fringe worn with long, layered waves that play up the cheekbones.

Wispy bangs and off-center parts will soften the square look of the face. Height at the crown will elongate your symmetrical shape. If your hair is straight, you may want to consider a body wave, as some curl or wave to the hair will achieve a nice balance to an angular facial shape.

Hair should either be long enough to cascade to the tops of the shoulders or, if shorter, should end either just above or below the jawline.

Avoid

Long straight styles can accentuate square jawbones. In styling, adding roundness to the face as well as some height at the crown, or wispy bangs, will have you on the beauty fast track.

FAMOUS FACES: SQUARE SHAPE

Square facial shapes include Demi Moore, Kristin Scott Thomas, Kyra Sedgwick, and Isabella Rosellini.

Rectangle

Rectangle faces are long and slender, about the same width at the forehead and just below the cheekbones. Faces may have a very narrow chin or a very high forehead.

Flattering

Short to medium-length hair is wonderful for the rectangle facial shape. By cutting the hair into a short or medium length, the outline of the cut will shorten the look of the length of the face.

Adding fullness at the sides will add width to the look. Wispy bangs will shorten the appearance of the length and balance the look of a long and slender face. Layers work well with the straight lines in your face.

Avoid

Wearing tresses long and stick-straight will add unwanted length to the face. When the hair gets past the shoulders, it will drag your face down to appear even longer. Center parts are too angular—a side part or zigzag part is much more fun and flattering.

FAMOUS FACES: RECTANGLE SHAPE

Some celebrities with a rectangle facial shape are Gwyneth Paltrow, Kirstie Alley, Janet Jackson, Niki Taylor, Jessica Simpson, and Stephanie Seymour.

Diamond/Triangle

Diamond/triangle faces are the reverse of the heart shape—a dominant jawline with narrowing at the cheek bones and temples.

Flattering

Select styles that add softness and width at the cheekbones and fill out a pointed chin. Hairstyles that utilize sleek side panels to slim the wide cheekbones are beautiful on this facial shape.

Shorter hair balances the prominent jawline. Styles that are full at the temples and taper at the jaw will allow your facial shape to shine. By wearing styles that are full at the temples and taper at the jawline, you achieve a balance that can be pretty and feminine, allowing understated features to be accented.

Off-center parts, wedges, and shag looks work for you very well. Lots and lots of layers will help achieve fullness through the upper part of the face. Try tucking your hair behind your ears, as this will draw attention to your eyes and add width to this area.

Long, full hairstyles draw attention to the jawline. If you go with long hair, it should be kept tight at the nape. Center parts are too severe for the triangular facial shape.

Too much height at the crown of the head should be avoided. You will want to stay away from putting most of the weight of your haircut at the jawline and below. This will give the appearance of added weight to the face.

FAMOUS FACES: DIAMOND/TRIANGLE SHAPE

Faces in the spotlight with diamond/triangle facial shapes include Kathy Ireland and Sandra Bullock.

Pear/Inverted Heart

This shape is widest at the jawline, with graduated narrowing upward from the cheeks to the forehead.

Flattering

Add width to the top half of the pear/inverted heart facial shape by adding carefully constructed texture extending from the cheeks upward toward the top of the crown. Pear/inverted heart shapes are great candidates to experiment in adding soft height in the crown area while keeping the hair closer to the sides from the cheeks onward. Bangs of all lengths—be it wispy or full-blown bangs—are very complimentary to the pear/inverted heart facial shape.

Avoid

Chin-length 'dos will create wideness in the fullest part of the face. Swept-forward hairstyles will add too much "weight" at the already generous cheeks and chin areas. Hair that is too short will not be as flattering as hair that is longer and free flowing, creating a visual line to slim the face and chin.

WHAT ABOUT BOB?

One style that seems to never go out of style and, believe it or not, can work for all of the facial shapes—not just the perfect oval face—is the bob. It takes the great eye of a fabulous stylist to find the perfect bob for your facial shape. Here are some tips for creating the ever-hot bob:

- To make a thin or rectangular face look fuller, try a chin-length bob with bangs and longer layers in the back. Faces generally look fuller with symmetrical styles and longer side fringes.
- To slim excessive width at the cheekbones, select a bob that uses sleek layered front hair panels that are cut to minimize the cheeks.
- To slim a round face, go with a side-parted bob cut below the chin with choppy or shaggy layers.
- To soften a square jaw and wide chin, opt for a shorter cut that ends at the nape of the neck and is carefully layered in front to avoid bulk at the chin.

THE RIGHT HAIRSTYLE FOR YOUR LIFESTYLE

While knowing your face shape is the perfect starting point for getting a great haircut, you'll also need to look at certain aspects of your lifestyle to avoid costly haircut fixes. You should also factor:

- Hair's texture—be it straight, curly, or wavy
- Age
- Lifestyle
- Facial features that you wish to highlight—or minimize

While you might have your mind and your heart set on a style, if the style is not compatible with the texture of your hair, you might be spending all of your free time in front of the mirror wrestling with styling products, hot rollers, curling irons, flat-irons, etc., just to keep something of the 'do that you dreamed of. Whew! I can think of better ways to spend in front of the mirror—like enjoying a style that both works for you *and* on you.

Top to Bottom

Tall gals and girls with lots of texture and/or full tresses should skip the super-short chops or crop hairstyles. Petite women should forego hairstyles that overwhelm their delicate features or contrast with their overall body shape.

The Right Coif for Your Age

While it is true that "you are only as young as you feel," hairstyles that are obviously created for a much younger or older crowd will not be as flattering as a style that matches who you are—where you are—in this life stage.

THRIFTY TIP

Trying a super-young style will probably not actually make you look younger; in fact, it will make you look older, as you appear to be trying to capture your lost youth. So save your money and find a better style for you now!

The same goes for young women trying hairstyles that are designed for the mature woman. Instead of making you look sophisticated, you will look matronly—not a good thing.

Wash and Go?

Lifestyles have a lot to do with hairstyles. If you absolutely, positively, have to be out of bed and on the road for work each morning in fifteen minutes or less, hairstyles requiring anything but a blow-dry-and-go routine will not work for you. Just setting up and heating up all of the things needed for a high maintenance hairstyle on a short time budget will make you as nervous as having too much coffee!

On the other hand, practice makes perfect, and once you get the hang of what is needed to create your dream hairstyle, you can quite easily multitask your morning, shaving moments off here and there. After all, aren't we women the queens of multi-tasking?

IF YOU GOT IT, FLAUNT IT. IF YOU HAVE TOO MUCH, HIDE IT!

Your individual facial features are what make you you. As with the different facial shapes, knowing what to highlight and what to minimize with facial features helps maximize beauty, creating the most flattering look for you.

LONG FOREHEAD: Bangs, bangs, bangs. Besides downplaying a forehead, bangs can slim a round face, soften sharp edges, and play up beautiful eyes.

SHORT FOREHEAD: Choose styles that are worn away from the face and styles that add interest elsewhere, such as a flip at the ears, or soft cascading curls on the top of the shoulders.

PROMINENT NOSE: Hair that is upswept and off the face or softened with carefully designed bangs will balance the face beautifully.

CLOSE-SET EYES: Hairstyles that go forward on the sides will create a farther-away eye look. Adding texture will also create interest and illusion.

WIDE-SET EYES: To balance eye width, avoid lots of texture or volume along the sides. Hair that is pulled away gives the impression of perfectly proportioned eyes.

DOUBLE CHIN: Slim a double chin by selecting a long, choppy shag style with layers that softly curve in toward the chin and down along the neck.

NO CHIN: Maximize a nonexistent or small chin with a short, blunt bob that opens up and highlights the area.

SMALL MOUTH: Maximize a small mouth with a shorter angled bob or blunt cut to draw the line of the face inward and minimize the jaw.

PROMINENT MOUTH: Minimize a prominent mouth with longer sweeping styles that softly frame the face and draw attention to the eyes.

When dealing with what you consider a "problem" feature, remember that we are most critical of ourselves, and in most cases, we are the only ones who consider it to be a challenge in the first place. Rather than focusing on any facial shortcomings or facial shape concerns, turn your attention to maximizing your best features and being your most glamorous, glorious best!

THE LONG AND THE SHORT OF IT

How do you think your favorite star's hair goes from short in one photo to long in another? Hair extensions. Hair extensions are literally bonded to the real hair with heat for a look that is as natural as can be. Once the hair extensions are in place, you can wash, brush, and style the hair as usual. On average, extensions last about three to four months. They can, however, be removed, should you change your mind before then. Although hair extensions are pretty pricey, to some the cost of having long hair in just one afternoon is worth it.

Find the most flattering stylist who will take into consideration all of the factors that make a great hairdo. Together you and your stylist can find the perfect 'do for you. And if the stylist is smart, he or she will show you exactly how to create your glamour girl look—every day, and not just on hair appointment day. After all, you are a walking, talking, billboard for the stylist's work. How great is it to have a real glamour girl sporting one's handiwork?!

Chapter Three

High Styling

" Another thing about women is that they can be persuaded to do anything with their hair, except leave it alone. "

—UNKNOWN

F inding the best (affordable) stylist can be a bit tricky, but with a little knowledge and a bit of know-how you can find the stylist of your dreams, without the nightmare prices.

Highly acclaimed celebrity hairdressers such as Jonathan and Nicky Clarke can command and *get* anywhere from $400 to $700 for just a haircut. But hold on—this chapter is all about finding the right stylist for you, working with the size of your budget—not your mortgage payment!

MAKE IT LAST

When visiting a new stylist, call ahead and book a complimentary consultation. Try to book the appointment for the very end of his or her scheduled shift. By having the last appointment, you will not be rushed because of the next client. You will have time to ask all of your questions, and the stylist will have time to answer them all. Now that's a lasting impression!

There are many oh-so-fabulous hairstylists who work in the real world and for a lot less. The key to finding these talented and affordable stylists is to take your time and do a little homework.

STYLE SLEUTH

Here are some sly ways to find the best stylist for your budget:

CHECK OUT NATIONAL HAIRSTYLING TRAINING SCHOOLS. National brands such as Redken, Matrix, or John Paul Mitchell have schools where highly trained stylists and educators travel to supervise hair services at local beauty schools around the country. Some of the schools offer days that are open to the public. Contact the beauty school in your area to see if it participates in national trainer visits.

SEE IF YOU CAN SCHEDULE AN APPOINTMENT WITH AN APPRENTICE. Most high-end salons have apprentices to a master hairstylist. Famous stylists to the stars had to start somewhere. Most of the great stylists have at least one and sometimes several apprentices who have exceptional training and skills. The difference? The apprentices, who are there to learn from the masters, charge less—sometimes up to 75 percent less. When you book with a master's apprentice, you can be sure that you will get the highest of quality design, at a down-to-earth price.

SEARCH FOR HAIRSTYLISTS WHO WORK IN DAY SPAS RATHER THAN HAIR SALONS. Spas will often offer package deals that allow you to get frequent-visitor discounts or even free services when you purchase a number of treatments. Some day spa packages include a complimentary haircut and style.

CHECK YOUR LOCAL PAPER FOR ANNOUNCEMENTS OF NEW SALONS OR DAY SPAS (WITH HAIR SERVICES). Many times they will offer grand opening specials on services and products. Why not swing by one during the grand opening, and ask for a tour of the facilities? The staff will be happy to show you around. If your schedule permits it, hang around and see what the stylists are doing, and whom you think you might like to schedule a consultation with. Consultations *should* be free—but always ask. Also, ask the staff who they think would be the best stylist for the look you have in mind.

INQUIRE IF THE SALON YOU ARE LOOKING INTO OFFERS BUNDLING SERVICES. Bundling is where you schedule your hair color or highlight, cut, and styling at the same time. Often, the salon will discount the complete service when booked together.

SEE IF THE SALON OFFERS "EARLY BIRD" SPECIALS FOR EARLIER IN THE WEEK, OR PERHAPS DURING THE MORNING HOURS, WHEN THE SALON IS NOT AS BUSY. Traditionally the front part of the week is slower than Thursdays, Fridays, and, of course, Saturdays.

CHECK FOR THE "BOOTH RENTERS." A booth renter is a term used for a stylist who rents space from a salon without actually being an employee. Booth renters are self-employed, set their own rates for services, and may be willing to negotiate a package deal. Some independent stylists will also give discounts for ongoing referrals. Others may trade a complimentary haircut for a certain number of referrals.

CHECK OUT THE SALON AND DAY SPA WEB SITES. Often "subscribers" get special offerings as a thank you for signing up. Most offer "daily e-mail specials" in which the salon or spa looks at the next day's bookings and offers a discount to fill the book. It is usually 20 to 30 percent off the regular price. So if you can escape on short notice, you can get a great new you on sale!

ASK, ASK, ASK. Friends and family all have to go to the salon—ask whom they know. If you see a hairstyle that you love on a person—stranger or not—ask the person where she gets her hair done. We all love getting a compliment, and, even more, love sharing if it was a good deal!

HOW TO TELL YOUR STYLIST WHAT YOU WANT

Again, the more homework you do up front, the more likely the chance that you'll love your haircut on the first try! Once you find a stylist, use these tips to help you help your hairstylist understand your dream style.

- Do your stylist sleuthing before you visit your stylist so that you have a solid understanding of your hair goals.
- If you wear glasses, remember to bring them to the salon when meeting with your new stylist, so that he or she can take the frames into consideration when deciding on an overall style.
- Another tip for the girls who wear glasses: Try to choose frames and a hairstyle that compliment each other. Large frames could spoil a neat, feathery cut, and very fine frames could be overpowered by a large, voluminous style. Ask your stylist for suggestions before you have your next eye doctor's appointment.
- A picture is truly worth a thousand words. Bring in clear, consistent photos that show your desired hairstyle in as many positions and angles as possible. Select models who resemble your personal facial shape, body shape, length of neck, and hair texture.
- To show your desired hair color, again, photos are the ticket. If not photos, then bring in swatches of the color (or colors) that you desire. Remember, what you see as Ravishing Red may be Flaming Orange to someone else.
- Be open to listening to the stylist's feedback. Hear him or her out. You have the right to not to opt for that direction, but if you are willing to listen, he or she will be more likely to listen to you. Stylists are the experts, so usually

compromise gets the look that you want with the ease of care that you need.

- When stylists say that they get what look you are trying to achieve, ask them to repeat it back to you. If what they repeat is a bit off, restate what you want and give further instructions. Ask them to repeat it again. When *they* get it, *you* will get your dream look.

- Pay attention. Once the stylist begins to work on your hair, keep your eyes open and pay attention. If he or she seems to veer off course, be prepared to politely stop, and explain again what you are looking for. By all means, do not wait until it is too late!

We shampoo, blow-dry, cut, color, crimp, braid, curl, flat-iron, style, and straighten our crowning glory on a daily basis. How you feel about your hair has a dramatic effect on your day and your mood. When it is a wonderful hair day, it shows—all is right with the world. Have a bad hair day and, well, I bet you know the rest of the story. Decide here and now to banish bad hair days forever and opt for only glorious, glamour girl days from here on out.

Chapter Four

The Cutting Edge

" There are at least fifty ways of cutting fringes, from the Cleopatra block to Claudia Schiffer's wisps. There is a fringe just waiting for you! "

—NICKY CLARKE, INTERNATIONAL HAIRSTYLIST

A good haircut can make you feel fantastic. Having perfect glamorous tresses increases your confidence, makes you feel sexier and more powerful, and can even make you feel taller and thinner! Most important, a good haircut should reflect your personality. Styled in the right way, a haircut can even act as an instant facelift, helping to minimize attention from areas of the face that are beginning to show signs of aging, and instead highlight your most flattering features such as great cheekbones or beautiful eyes. Quite simply, a good cut will give your entire look a new lease on life.

THRIFTY TIP

Hair is usually the first thing to be altered when a woman is making a major life change. Be it a new career, or the beginning (or the end) of a relationship, something about changing hairstyles signals (at least in our own minds, anyway) that something or someone new is on the horizon.

A visit to the salon for a bit of pampering or reinventing has been known to banish many a bad mood. It seems that once you've found the right hairstyle, everything else falls into place with regard to your overall look.

In Chapter Three, I gave you pointers on how to choose the best stylist for your needs. Once you have selected your stylist, schedule a consultation to talk about your hair and the style or cut that you want. Let he or she walk you through what she plans to do to your hair. Ask about upkeep—that is, how often to schedule a cut and what products are recommended to keep the look and condition. Don't be afraid to say that you are on a beauty budget and would like to know which products are totally necessary and which you can economize with. It could be that your drugstore shampoo and conditioner are just fine and that you just need to add some salon sculpting gel in order to achieve the "salon" look.

CUTTING CONSIDERATIONS

Whatever the reason and whatever the style, the important thing is to maintain the mane by scheduling an appointment for at least a trim every six to eight weeks to avoid split ends and help maintain condition and manageability.

IF ONLY ONCE

If you can possibility swing it budgetwise, decide to splurge on a truly great, trendy, high-end salon for a consultation and cut. You can enjoy "living the high life" long after the experience is over. Be sure to take photos of your hair from the front, sides, and back as soon as you leave the salon. When it is time for a trim, take the photos to your regular stylist so he or she can see the style and re-create it—for a much more reasonable price. Don't worry that your stylist will think that you "cheated" on him or her. Most likely, the stylist will be excited to hear all about your uptown experience. He or she will want the details about what you saw, how the salon looks, and what other people were doing.

The hair on the head grows at different rates in different places, so a haircut can get out of shape within a few weeks. For a very short stylish cut, the hair might need tidying up every four weeks. If you are trying to grow your hair long, then a trim every three months may be sufficient.

Work with What You Have

Be realistic. How much time do you really want to spend on your hair every day? Also, how much time do you have, realistically?

If you choose a hairstyle that takes fifteen minutes in the morning and you can only spare ten minutes, you will not be happy nor will you get the look that you want—no matter how much you multitask.

Whether your hair is straight or curly, dark or blonde, wavy or wispy, if you try to alter your natural hair to the extreme, you most likely will end up compromising on the condition of your hair and being a slave to your high-maintenance look. This is not glamorous by any means!

Ask the stylist to show you two or three different ways that you can wear your hair with your new style. Experiment with the new learned ways to wear your hair. After all, remember: You do not wear the same outfit every day, so why should you have the same hairstyle day in and day out?

THE LONG AND THE SHORT OF IT

Trying to figure out what length will work best for you. This section can help steer you in the right direction.

Long Hair

Long hair is often considered to be the most feminine, romantic, and, of course, a favorite with the opposite sex. To keep the counterculture "hippie" style from hitting your scene, keep the locks in excellent condition and go for a layered cut. A layered cut will add shape around the face and give a defined style. With well-shaped layers, hair will not fall too heavily across the face, but rather move and outline the face beautifully.

Middle of the Road

Mid-length hairstyles are one of the most popular, because they give the illusion of length and can flow and wave, but may also be trimmed regularly. Mid-length styles are a bit easier to care for as they offer greater variety in terms of different cuts, and it is easy to change your hairstyle. You can wear your hair up in a glamorous French twist for an evening out, and the next day, pull it back in the ever popular ponytail.

Short Hair

Feminine and hip, short hair can be downright sexy. It is a wonderful option for women who want a feminine image mixed with a strong sense of self. Short hairstyles can quickly create a personal signature look for the wearer—think Meg Ryan and Pink. Short, sassy, sexy styles are definitely glamorous when layers are added to define texture and volume, giving the hair greater depth and making styling simple and fun.

HAIRDRESSER-SPEAK

It can be a bit intimidating when your stylist starts throwing around hairdressing lingo. Here's a cheat sheet to help level the playing field.

LAYERING: Hair is thinned and tapered to create a layered look. Hair may be layered in to make the longer part on the outside or on the inside. With layering, hair may be cut to create many different effects.

CHOPPY: This describes hair that has been cut using a texturizing method such as a razor to create a choppy finish to the hair.

TEXTURIZING: This method of cutting uses tools such as a razor, clippers, or texturizing scissors. Texturizing scissors are like regular cutting scissors, but one blade is serrated, enabling the stylist to reduce hair weight evenly throughout the cut.

FEATHERING: Instead of using scissors to cut the hair, a razor is used. A razor gives much more random cuts and finish, leaving the hair more disheveled and funky looking.

FLICK-OUTS: This method involves blow-drying the hair so that it flicks outward at the ends, creating volume and width. This a nice alternative to the more traditional look of blow-drying the hair under.

VOLUME: To build hair and add lift, volume can be temporary when done with styling products, or long lasting when done with a permanent wave before styling.

TAPERING: Extra hair bulk is removed and thins it, as well as removes length. Tapering enables the hair to curl more readily and encourages any natural wave in the hair.

THINNING: The extra weight of the hair is removed, but not the length. Thinning can help overly thick hair get the lift or curl that the style requires as it reduces excess hair weight.

CLUB CUTTING: This is a method of cutting the hair straight across, removing the length but retaining the bulk. It tends to discourage curling and is best used on straight hair. Club cutting is quite a skill, because while the hair is straight, the shape of head is not, and the way that the hair hangs will affect its length.

It seems that there is always a moment—that firm feeling that you get when you know you are ready for a new look. Logic seldom plays a part in this quest for more glamour. It is often a subconscious feeling more than a logical one. One day you look in the mirror and decide that the time is right.

BANG-BANG

If you decide to let your bangs grow out, have your stylist add a few long layers around the face. The bangs will blend in better as they are growing out. Also, a bit of highlights around the face adds drama and cache, making the growing-out part more fun.

Practically speaking, taking "a little off the top" or the sides or the bottom or wherever has a lot going for it. It boosts the hair's condition, whatever type you have, gives movement and bounce, and makes it easier to maintain. But, as they say, timing is everything. It is not in your—or your hair's—best interest to try a brand-new style and cut the day before you have something important going on. Instead, schedule your appointment a week or two before so that if something goes wrong, you have a chance to do something about it. You will also be able to work with the new style and capture the essence of what is necessary to re-create it on a daily basis.

Chapter Five

Thirty Thrifty Tips for Glamorous Hair

" A woman with her hair turned up always looks as if she were going some place—either the opera or the bath. "

—ORSON WELLES

Here are thirty instant tips that will give you Glamour Girl Hair—at Thrifty Girl price.

1. Shampoos and conditioners designed for different hair colors contain ingredients that will extend and enhance your hair color. Plus, most contain shine boosters for a bit of added pizzazz.

2. If you have medium-length or long hair, sleep with your hair loosely tied in a top of the head ponytail or bun. This will keep the wild hairs at bay, allowing for ease in the morning routine. Simply shake and comb it, rub a smoothing serum over the top layers, and give it a quick blast with the medium setting on the blow-dryer. Finish with a dash of hair spray and ta-da! You are done.

3. Refresh hair instantly and eliminate smoke and cooking smells by spritzing your favorite fragrance on a hairbrush and brushing it through your hair.

4. Hair masks are wonderful ways to bring hair back to life. Masks add shine, texture, and softness. Try to add one to your bathing routine once every couple of weeks. Shampoo, apply, and for the next couple of minutes while it is processing, why not exfoliate your body with some scented bath salts? Two beauty treatments in under two minutes—now that's beauty on the fast track!

5. Give short hair a midday pick-me-up by misting it with water and working a little styling product through from the roots to the ends.

6. When using a blow-dryer, switch to the cooler setting for the last minute or so. Applying too much heat at the scalp and neck can cause you to perspire and your hair to lose a little of its volume.

7. A deep side part is a quick way to get a sassy and sexy look.

8. For a change and quick update to your look, try a zigzag part of the hair. Instead of a straight line, a zigzag part looks fresh, fun, and—as an extra bonus—the crisscrossing of the part helps hide a needed color touch-up!

9. If your medium- or longer length hair decides to take the flat track, spray on some root volumizer and create a little lift by blow-drying the roots upside down. Finish with a spritz of hairspray to maintain the volume.

10. Scout around for tiny hair clips or barrettes that are the same color as your hair. Keep a few in your bag or desk drawer for those times when it seems as if each wisp of hair is on the escape. By matching your hair color, they blend in, making them less noticeable.

11. Wear a great pair of sunglasses on top of your head for an à la Audrey Hepburn look.

12. Baseball caps can be oh so chic when paired with a great pair of earrings and the perfect lip color. Look for hats with glitzy fabrics such as metallic or colored leather. They're perfect for the mad Saturday morning errand dashes.

13. Shampooing every day can dry hair out, so give it a rest with a couple of days off. It will not only save you time, but it will save your shine and condition. Instead of your normal shampoo, rinse with a refreshing blast of cool water, and then spritz your damp hair with a tiny bit of leave-in conditioner. Consider it a weekend off for your hair.

14. Dinner party ideas for hair: Long hair pulled back in a loose bun held in place with two chopstick-style hair accessories is a great way to look polished. Medium-length hair pulled in an asymmetrical side sweep secured with a festive barrette looks very glamorous. Short hair can look suave by slicking back the hair with a light application of pomade.

15. For outdoor winter activities, beat the hat head at its own game. Long hair can be sprayed with a light coating of leave-in conditioner and slicked back into a ponytail. Gals with short hair can use a moisturizing gel and comb the hair back as well. The hat is going to mash the hair down, anyway—at least this way your look is intentional and under your control.

16. Scarves radiate glamour. Long hair pulled back in a ponytail and tied with a colorful scarf adds a European flair to your look. Short-haired girls can simply wrap a scarf around the head and tie it in the back. You are now ready for that convertible cruise or scooter ride around town.

17. If your bob has become a bouffant, an instant rescue is to put a silk scarf tightly over the head and tie at the neck—just for just a minute or two. The scarf will de-puff the bouffant and bring back the bob. For really tough cases, you might have to keep on the scarf a couple of extra minutes. The scarf trick is also great to add sleekness to your style, as it smoothes down the hair cuticles and makes the hair shinier.

18. If you wake up to bed hair every morning, try changing your pillowcase to satin instead of cotton. Satin pillowcases allow the hair to slide across the pillow gently as you move in your sleep. Cotton, on the other hand, can cause friction and stress the hair. Another beauty bonus is that satin pillowcases will keep your face from creasing if you tend to press your face into the pillow.

19. For some easy curls, try taking a random 1- to 2-inch section of damp hair, twist the strand tightly, and secure in place with a clip. Let the hair dry naturally, only taking it down when the hair is completely dry. Don't comb it, but instead turn your head upside down and use your fingers to gently comb through it to break up the curl. Spray and go.

20. Flyaway hair can be quickly tamed by taking a cloth sprayed with an antistatic spray and gently rub over the top layer of the hair. Try not to comb, as the flyaways could return.

21. If you are setting your hair before a bath or shower, close the bathroom door so that the steam does not escape. Spray your hair with a light setting spray and roll your hair as usual. The steam will help set the curls. Remove the rollers when your hair is completely dry. Simply run your fingers through the hair to style. Finish with a dash of hair spray.

22. Baby powder is a great hair volumizer. For days when your hair has flattened, sprinkle a little baby powder on your roots, flip your hair upside down and gently shake the hair with your fingers to distribute the powder down the hair shaft. Stand up and spritz the hair with a style-setting hair spray.

23. Try partially drying your hair before applying styling products. By drying the hair a bit first, you will be able to use less product and save time drying the hair as well. Totally wet hair can also dilute product effectiveness, causing the hair to go flat or lose the style more quickly.

24. Revitalize dull locks by shampooing once or twice a month with a detoxifying shampoo that will remove any built-up residue in the hair. Follow with a deep conditioning treatment and marvel at the wonderful difference it makes. A quick and thrifty tip is to make your own detoxifying shampoo by putting some of your regular shampoo in a separate bottle and adding a couple of aspirin to effectively remove excesses from the hair. An easy way to add a deep condition to your regular conditioner is to squeeze a couple of vitamin E capsules into it.

25. Poor rinsing is one of the prime causes of dull hair. A good remedy—just rinse your hair twice as long as you think that you need to.

26. Rinsing hair with champagne brings out blonde highlights. Conditioning the hair with another adult beverage, beer, adds a lot of shine to your hair. So the next time you raise a glass, save a little extra for your hair.

27. Beach hair can be pretty if done right. If your hair is medium to long and you take a dip in the sea, make two or more braids after coming out of the water. Allow to completely dry. After drying, take out the braids, and run your fingers through the hair to create sassy and sexy wavy hair. If your hair is short, just scrunch it up with your fingers and allow to dry. You can achieve beach hair at home by putting two tablespoons of sea salt in a six-ounce spritzer. Wet your head completely and follow the braid or crunch instructions.

28. For really BHD (Bad Hair Days) when nothing will work, rather than fight it, join it. Pull your hair back using a wet comb. Add a little dab of conditioner to give your hair a bit of beauty treatment and staying power. Pick out a headband in your favorite color and put it on. Your hair will be out of your face and off your mind. Plus, now it looks like it was your plan all along.

29. Give your styling tools a good soaking. Every month soak your hairbrush, comb, and styling accessories in hot water and some buildup-removing shampoo for two to three minutes. Rinse and clean out hair with a comb. Allow to dry.

30. For glamorous hair accessories, look no further than your jewelry box. Rings can dress up hair ties. Clip-on earrings can be used as focal points in an updo. A necklace can double as a headband. Dressy pins can be wonderful barrettes; just use a bobby pin or two to secure.

PART 2

THE
THRIFTY
GIRL'S
GUIDE TO
GLAMOROUS
SKIN

This next section is devoted to the skin you're in. I'll show you how to do the best at-home facial, how to do your makeup—from the office to the opera—and how to tame those crazy brows. I'll cover it all, and help you appreciate your own beautiful skin.

Chapter Six

Let's Face It

<blockquote>
“ There are no ugly women,

only lazy ones. ”

—HELENA RUBINSTEIN
</blockquote>

You could not be more up close and personal than you are with your skin—after all, you're covered with it! And while you can cover your skin with clothing, your face is always exposed and is what you see in the mirror each and every time you look. Facial skin tells the world your story. It reveals the quality of life and tells the tales of summers spent in the sun, late nights, sleeping in makeup, too much caffeine, and not enough water. But when you turn the other cheek, skin can reveal a soft glow, luminosity, a twinkle in the eye, and a healthy outlook on life.

GOOD NIGHT

Not getting enough sleep is known for causing physical symptoms, but lack of sleep also inhibits the immune system's ability to fight off viruses and bacteria that can cause pimples and acne. As we sleep, our entire body is going about the business of repairing itself. Our skin does most of its repairs between the hours of 1 and 4 A.M. Lack of sleep during this cell-rejuvenating time can trigger stress that causes the skin to look dull, tired, puffy, or sallow. Even worse—you wake up with a breakout! Remember, it is called "beauty sleep" for a reason. Get your z-z-z-z-s!

Even if, right now, at this minute, you are not in love with your skin, the good news is that skin is full of wonderfully, forgiving, and grateful cells that are excited to be paid even a little bit of attention and will respond quickly when handled with care. There is nothing like a little healthy vanity to motivate you to take care of your skin—is there?

The starting point to great skin is identifying what kind of skin you have. Modern skin care technology has evolved from just the dry, normal, oily, and combination skin types to now include subcategory conditions that affect the skin such as sensitivity, dullness, fine lines, irritation, and general pore size and condition.

Your skin can change from type to type and back again. It can also suffer from different conditions depending on your lifestyle, stress (good and bad), hormones, and even the climate. The key point to remember is that your skin can change at a moment's notice.

THRIFTY TIP

Just as you adjust your clothing based on the weather conditions, adjust your skin care routine based on your skin condition at the given moment. Thankfully, adapting to your current skin condition as it changes does not require a complete new skin care regime. So don't go out and buy all new products—maybe just a tweak here and there.

Think of it as putting on a scarf and gloves one day and a raincoat the next, depending on the environment.

SKIN TYPES AND REMEDIES

Not sure of your skin type? This section will help you determine your skin type, which should dictate what kind of products you use.

Dry Skin

The look of dry skin is tight, dull, and flaky. This is due to the lack of oil (sebum) in the skin. Dry skin chaps most quickly in the sun, wind, and cold. Dry skin can make you look older than what your driver's license says, if it is not respected. Dry skin can be confused with dehydrated skin; however, the key difference is that skin lacking surface moisture, like dehydrated skin, will respond in kind quickly when moisturizer is applied and water is consumed. True dry skin will still feel like it is missing something—wanting more.

Regime Remedy

Choose an extra-creamy cleanser and a toner without alcohol. Moisturizer should be thicker and more concentrated than moisturizers designed for normal or oily skin. Exfoliate the skin gently with a skin polisher once a week. This skin type benefits greatly from a facial mask that both hydrates and removes excess dead skin cells on a biweekly basis. Removing the dead skin cells allows skin care products to reach the deeper layers of the skin. Don't forget to drink lots of water.

Dehydrated Skin

Any skin type can develop dehydrated skin—even oily skins! Dehydrated skin is caused by overexposure to the weather elements (hot or cold), stress, illness, lack of water consumption, and controlled environments (indoor heat and A/C). Dehydrated skin looks and feels taut and dull, and may even itch.

Regime Remedy

Adding hydration gives this skin immediate relief. Drinking water while limiting caffeine does wonders for dehydrated skin types. Also, adding a moisturizer filled with water-loving ingredients such as humectants will give this parched skin a much needed "drink of water" to the skin. A moisturizing facial mask is a quick fix for putting water back into the skin. Choose cleansers and toners that are gentle and without alcohol.

Normal Skin

In this case, normal means perfect—the type of skin that we all would love to have. Normal skin has pH balance, allowing a skin texture that is neither oily nor dry. And as an added bonus, normal skin enjoys fewer breakouts. Lucky gals!

The phrase "keep it simple" was made for normal skin types. Cleanse with a water-based cleanser that rinses off easily, and follow with a mild toner. Moisturize lightly. Weekly maintenance includes a quick sloughing of dead skin cells with an exfoliator and occasional facial mask to keep this very envious skin type at its best.

Oily Skin

Slick, shiny, and at times greasy best describes oily skin. The pores look more open and, unfortunately, blackheads are almost standard with oily skins. The good news is that oily skins, rich with sebum, will wrinkle less; the bad news is the unpredictable breakouts, for one thing!

Regime Remedy

Skin care product choice is very important and can make a huge difference with oily skin. Surface oil can attract dirt and grime, causing the pores to become clogged. This skin type must, without a doubt, be kept clean while at the same time not overstripped. In fact, cleaning with overzealous products will actually cause the skin to produce more oil—which is exactly what this skin does not need. Look for products that effectively remove oil while taking care of the skin. In other words, baby your oily skin. When a blemish happens, treat with a blemish-fighting ingredient such as benzoyl peroxide on the blemish culprit—not the entire face.

Combination Skin

This skin has a split personality. One part is in search of oil and the other wishing for drier days. The term "T-Zone" describes this skin to a T. In most cases, the forehead, nose and chin are oily while the cheeks and the eye area are as dry as dust.

Regime Remedy

The juggling act for combination skin is to keep the oil to a minimum while hydrating the dryer parts. Look for a cleanser and toner designed for combination skin. The moisturizer should be water-based and contain lots of hydrating properties to soothe the skin while protecting it. Exfoliate the skin at least once a week. For optimum skin, combine two different facial masks: one designed for oily skins on the forehead, nose, and chin, and a mask designed for dry and normal skins for the cheeks and eye areas.

Aging Skin

Chronologically, our skin is another day older each and every day. However, the skin can age environmentally and hormonally as well. Environmental aging occurs when the skin is over-exposed to the elements such as sunlight, controlled heat and air conditioning, and pollutants. The skin reacts by becoming drier, spotty, and flaky. Hormonal aging results from changes in hormones causing the skin to lose firmness and elasticity.

Regime Remedy

Use of a sunscreen is imperative. Almost 75 percent of premature aging is due to overexposure to the sun. Creams with anti-aging ingredients and products with firming properties will help repair and protect the skin from damage. Using products with AHA (alpha hydroxy acid) will increase skin cell production and elimination of dead cells.

Stressed Skin

Stressed skin takes on many faces, almost like the movie *Sybil*. A dead giveaway is skin that is flaky, blotchy, and blemish prone. Any and all skin types can be stressed, given the right circumstances. Common stressed-skin-producing elements are anxiety, pollution, harsh weather, and lack of sleep.

Regime Remedy

When choosing skin care products, look for words such as "soothing," "comforting," or "relaxing." Cleansers and toners need to be gentle. Mild and water-based moisturizers are the perfect response to soothe stressed skin. The skin will relax and rehydrate the skin at the same time.

Sensitive Skin

Each year more and more skins are reported to be sensitive—in fact, so much so that cosmetic companies are launching skin care lines especially designed for sensitive skins. Many beauty experts believe that the increase in cases of sensitive skin is due to lifestyle, illnesses, stress, allergy, and harsh products causing a reaction to the skin surface. Reactions include redness, itching, swelling, roughness of skin texture, or a feeling of burning.

Regime Remedy

To rule out an ingredient allergy, schedule an appointment with a dermatologist. All products used on the face should be mild and contain as few ingredients as possible. The most common irritants are fragrance, dyes, sunscreen, isopropyl alcohol, and benzoic acid. Introduce only one new product to the skin at a time. Allow the skin to adjust to the new product before adding another one to the regime. Look for the word "hypoallergenic" or labels that say "made for sensitive skin."

COOL, CALM, AND COLLECTED

If suddenly your skin is feeling sensitive due to chapping or irritation, calm it down with tea. Brew a pot of chamomile tea. Allow to cool, and pour into an ice cube tray. Freeze. Take out a frozen cube, wrap in cotton gauze, and rub gently around the face for five minutes. The skin will feel cool, calm and collected, and destressed.

You may discover that out of the eight skin types listed, your skin falls between two (or maybe even among three) different categories. Remember, just as you have changed over the years, so has your skin. Quite often, I meet with a client regarding her skin care regime, and she reports that although she has been using the same products for a few years, suddenly her skin is not responding, or maybe even now breaking out. I tell her that skin changes, too, and I bet she is not wearing the same clothes or driving the same car that she did when she first began using the product line—so why should her skin remain the same? Having beautiful skin is not revolutionary—it's evolutionary!

Chapter Seven

Caught on Tape

66 At 20 you have the skin God gave
you. At 40 you have the skin you
have purchased. And either way, at
60 you have the skin you deserve! 99

—COCO CHANEL

A fast and easy way to determine what condition your skin condition is in—and how your skin is aging—is to take the "caught on tape" test. This chapter will cover how to test your skin (no cheating!), and how to read the results.

THE TAPE TEST

First cleanse and tone the skin. Do not moisturize. Wait two hours to allow the skin to return to its normal state. Begin the skin test by placing six small strips of adhesive tape one at a time on the following areas of the face:

1. Begin with a strip of tape applied vertically on the center of the forehead from the scalp line down to the bridge of the nose (in between the brows).

2. Place another piece of tape on the outside corner of each eye (where the crow's feet would be).

3. The fourth and fifth tape strips are applied across the apple part of each cheek.

4. Finally, put a tape strip above the upper lip (like a moustache).

Gently press the tape strips onto the skin. Remove the tape one strip at a time, as you review the skin agers below:

CRINKLY AREAS RESEMBLING THIN LINES, SUCH AS ROADS ON A MAP, INDICATE DEHYDRATED SKIN— WHICH IS A SKIN LACKING IN SURFACE MOISTURE. As a note, however, these crinkly lines are good indicators of where your skin will wrinkle if left unchecked. Keeping a hydrating moisturizer on the skin, as well as misting the skin with a mineral water mist a couple of times a day, will help ease the crinkles and keep the wrinkles at bay.

FLAKES ON THE TAPE INDICATE DRY, DEAD SKIN CELLS. This condition is caused from not properly removing cleansing and/or makeup products, as well as not exfoliating the skin on a regular basis. Making a facial exfoliating product, such as a gentle skin polisher or a mask once or twice a week, depending on your skin type, part of your skin care regime will aid in reducing skin's flakiness. On a daily basis, using a clean, warm, moist, washcloth along with your facial cleanser will help with daily flake buildup.

LINES ARE AN INDICATION OF A REDUCTION OF COLLAGEN AND ELASTIN IN THE SKIN CELLS. Collagen and elastin are responsible for keeping the skin plump and firm. As we age, our bodies begin producing less of these important skin firmers, so our skin begins to sag and lose elasticity. To encourage younger looking skin, opt to add to your skin care product lineup a couple of high-performance products, with the terms "anti-aging" or "skin firming" in the product description.

VERTICAL LIP LINES ARE CAUSED FROM SUN DAMAGE, SMOKING, AND/OR PURSING THE LIPS. To reduce the appearance of the lip lines, add an application of your eye cream over the top of the lip area as part of your twice-a-day skin care regime. And when you catch yourself pursing your lips—stop it!

X MARKS THE SPOT. To determine if your skin is really sensitive, try this tip. With a clean thumbnail, gently make a light X between your eyebrows. If the redness remains for a while, your skin is sensitive in addition to your usual skin type.

Most of the skin conditions we have are a direct result of how we treat our skin. Exposure to the sun, sleeping in makeup, smoking, not drinking enough water and/or drinking excessive caffeine or alcohol, poor eating habits, and insufficient vitamins are all contributors to how we age.

H$_2$O U

Water, without a doubt, is the number one beauty product in the world. There is absolutely nothing that makes a bigger difference to your beauty life than H$_2$O. Water hydrates the skin, flushes toxins from the body, and keeps all of the systems working. If you are not drinking eight full glasses of this incredible beauty product each and every day, you are missing the beauty boat—and it shows.

While we cannot go back in time, we can certainly go forward with a good simple skin care regime that will only take two minutes in the morning and two minutes in the evening. So start now, and go as long as you're alive. Don't be the one who wakes up at fifty-something and says: "Wow, I should have worn an eye cream!" Surely a glamour girl's skin is worth four minutes a day!

BEAUTY SLEEP

Sleeping in makeup takes at least ten days off the life of your face. As you sleep, you toss and turn—grinding the makeup into the pores, pushing the grime and dirt deeper into the skin. Also, mascara left on the eyes causes the eyelashes to be bent and squished with the old cakey stuff, causing breakage. Before it's lights out, it's makeup off.

Chapter Eight

Skin Deep

" If you take care of your skin, your
skin, your complexion, will take
care of itself. "

—HELENA RUBINSTEIN

More advancement in skin care technology has happened between 1990 and the present than occurred from 1989 all the way back to the time of Cleopatra! It seems as if a new skin breakthrough is happening on a monthly, if not weekly, basis. Why all the concentration on skin care technology? In two words: baby boomers. We can (and should) thank the generation that is showing the world that aging is not going to be taken lightly—and certainly not without a fight!

But with all of the breakthroughs and "revolutionary" scientific findings—why aren't we in nirvana with our skin? In one word: confusion. Peptide this, and retinol that. No wonder we, as well as our skin, are confused. Who can pronounce the ingredient furfuryladenine? Although it *sounds* like a fungus you could get in the changing room of the gym, it is, believe it or not, used to fight fine lines and wrinkles and is also called kinetin.

While all of the fancy ingredients certainly help keep the skin looking and feeling its best, the key to beautiful, glamorous skin is simple and much easier to pronounce—and can even be inexpensive! The successful skin care formula is consistency—day in and evening out, with an easy-to-follow skin care regime.

BEAUTIFUL SKIN BASICS

The following are the essential components of a simple and effective skin regimen.

Cleansing

The first step to beautiful skin is cleansing the skin in the morning and again at night. Since the body is busily repairing itself while we sleep, the morning cleansing is just as important as removing a full face of makeup in the evening. Cleansing in the morning wakes up the skin as well as removes any pore debris and overnight skin cell elimination, allowing for a smoother makeup application.

The evening cleansing removes all of the makeup and day's exposure to the environment. Cleansing the skin at night literally "takes the day off" the face and prepares the skin for nighttime nourishment.

Cleansers can be rinse-off or tissue-off—whatever your personal preference. The consensus is that Americans like a rinse-off cleanser, and Europeans favor the kind that is taken off with tissues or cotton pads. The key word to cleansing and cleansers is *gentle*.

Wash the face in warm, not hot, water to loosen the debris from the pores and remove dead skin cells. Taking about a dime-size dab of cleanser, wet one hand and rub the hands together to spread the cleanser before applying to the face. Moving the hands in a light circular motion will increase blood circulation as the face is being cleansed. Cleanse for one minute in the morning and about two minutes in the evening (to ensure thoroughly removing makeup). Rinse with slightly cool water and pat dry. Always keep in mind, when bathing or washing your face, that too hot or too cold water can cause capillaries in your skin to break.

Toning

A toner's job is to remove any residual cleanser and regulate the skin's pH balance. To tone or not to tone—that is the beauty expert question. Some experts feel that oily skins can benefit from skin toning as the toner calms the skin, and tightens the pores. Some feel that dry skins, on the other hand, can do without a toner, as the dry skin does not need extra stimulation. While it is a personal choice, to me, cleansing the skin without toning is like putting the clothes from the washing machine to the dryer without rinsing! I believe that all skins can benefit from a toner, especially toning products containing essential oils designed to hydrate and soothe the skin. After all, toners are the first product left on the skin.

> ### HONEY, I SHRUNK MY FACE
> If after you have cleansed and toned your skin, your skin feels like it is too tight, you might have just shrunk it! The taut feeling is caused by the removal of all moisture from the skin, causing it to feel like it is overly tight and taut. Switch to products that will cleanse the skin without stripping it of all moisture, like a hydrating cleanser and toner.

After cleansing, apply a cotton pad (or mist the skin) with toner. Cover the entire face and neck. Allow to dry.

Moisturizing

Moisturizers are a barrier between you and the outside world. They are designed to envelop the skin with hydration while protecting your skin from the environment. Moisturizers come in several types, from lotion and creams to balms and gels. As a rule, the thicker the texture of a moisturizer, the more oil it has. The thinner the consistency, the more water the moisturizer contains.

Moisturizers should leave the skin feeling and looking dewy—not oily or greasy. Just as we lighten up our clothing when the seasons change, the same traditionally holds true for moisturizers. A rich and thick moisturizer feels wonderful on the skin when the weather outside is frightful. A thin coating of a moisturizing lotion as the season heats up will protect the skin without feeling like you have struck oil.

Following the instructions on the package, after toning the skin, apply the moisturizer to the face and neck with the finger pads. Gently pat into the skin.

Night Cream

While some skin types can get away with just one moisturizing product for both day and night, for most of us, night creams definitely deserve a place on the vanity table. There are proven differences in skin activity during the daytime as opposed to nighttime. During the night, as we sleep, the body is devoting itself to repairing and recovering from the day's activities. Night creams contain ingredients that over the course of the night penetrate and nourish the skin deeper than a daytime moisturizer can. Think of it as backing up your skin computer.

After cleansing and toning, apply night cream before going to bed. It is best to apply night cream about five to ten minutes before retiring, to allow the cream to penetrate the skin and not be rubbed off on your pillow.

Eye Cream

The skin around the eyes is less than one-quarter as thick as the rest of the facial skin. Also, this tender skin is lacking oil glands, consequently making the skin around the eyes much more delicate. Eye creams are especially designed for the eye area, as they contain milder ingredients and spread more easily than facial moisturizers.

After cleansing, toning, and moisturizing (day or night), apply a tiny bit of eye cream to the eye area using the ring finger to pat the cream into the skin. The ring finger applies the least amount of pressure, so patting will not pull this tender skin area. Gently massage in a clockwise circle around the lid and underneath the eye. Use any cream left over on the finger to apply to the top of the lip area to keep those pesky vertical lip wrinkles at bay.

SKINCARE EXTRAS

In addition to your everyday skin care regimen, here are some other steps you may want to add on a regular—but less often— basis.

Exfoliating

About every twenty-eight to forty days, depending on age and skin condition, the skin has a new layer of skin cells working upward toward the surface. As they emerge, the older skin cells are being sloughed off. To help remove the surface dead skin cells and allow the newer skin cells to linger longer, exfoliating the skin is a great way to give the skin an extra boost. Once the dead skin cells are removed, the plumper, smoother, and healthier skin cells make the skin appearance more radiant.

There are chemical and manual exfoliating products. Chemical solutions contain AHAs (alpha hydroxy acids) to remove the dead skin cells, while the manual exfoliators use scrubbing type materials to remove the surface dead skin.

Newer, more effective exfoliating products contain both manual and chemical ingredients. First, an exfoliating cleanser is used to remove the top layer of dead skin cells. Rinse it off and apply a chemical solution to the skin for a specified period of time (three to ten minutes, depending on the formula). Follow up with a toner to both remove the chemical product as well as prepare the skin for hydration.

Try these products—they work great and don't cost a fortune:

- Hello Beautiful Peel Kit
- Olay Regenerist Peel System

Exfoliators are one of those skin care extras, but in today's environmentally challenging times, they should be in your beauty basket of must-haves.

Masks

Facial masks are miracle workers for the skin. Masks can be gel, cream, peel-off, or clay. Made for just about every skin condition known, a mask is a great way to bring your skin back to life. While no esthetician would be without an array of masks for facials, finding a good one for you is easy, once you know the score. If your skin is oily, choose one designed to regulate oil production and rid the skin of surface toxins. If your skin is dry, try one designed to rehydrate the skin and put the moisture back into the skin cells. For combination skins, a couple of masks may be just what the beauty expert ordered. Choose a moisturizing one for the cheeks and eye areas, while applying an oily skin type mask for the forehead, nose, and chin.

Cleanse and tone the skin. Apply the appropriate mask and leave on the skin for the specified amount of time. Remove as directions indicate and follow with a moisturizer. For an instant pick-me-up, for the last five minutes that the mask is to be on the skin, lie down and put your head slightly off the side of the bed. This will increase blood flow to the skin's surface, allowing the mask's ingredients to work a little better. This is a wonderful preparty or night-out treatment, as your skin will glow.

I suggest trying these inexpensive masks:

- Biotherm Hydra-Detox Masque
- Olay Daily Facials Mask

Skin Brighteners

Sometimes the skin needs a little help. Skin brighteners contain ingredients such as hydroquinone, licorice, and glycolic acids that help lighten and brighten the skin.

Brighteners help fade sun spots; melesma (also known as the mask of pregnancy), which is darker skin pigments; and freckles. Used on a regular basis, the skin brightener will lighten these trouble spots and give the skin a more luminous look.

Skin Firmers

In the world of anti-aging, firming products are all the rage. They work by trapping water in the skin, making the skin appear more plump and minimizing the loss of elasticity. Think of a plum versus a prune. They are exactly the same fruit—one has water and the other does not.

Skin firmers are an excellent addition to your skin care regime if lack of elasticity and skin slackness is visible. To use, after cleansing and toning, apply the skin firmer before your moisturizer and then apply your eye cream.

Here are some reasonably priced skin firmers:

- Korres, Alpine Herbs Anti-Stress
- Olay Total Effects 7 Signs Serum

NATURAL VERSUS SCIENCE

Natural is not always better. While poison ivy is natural, you would not put it on your face. Science has worked very hard to create products that last longer, keep bacteria to a minimum, and aid in further penetration of all ingredients—natural ones included. Science and nature need to work together to be in harmony.

What a great time to be a thrifty girl! With all of the skin care technology advancements happening as we speak, and competition between skin care companies, getting great ingredients at an even better price is as simple as reading the label. Remember, you only have one face—make it beautiful!

THE THRIFTY GIRL'S GUIDE TO A FABULOUS AT-HOME FACIAL

It has been said that beauty begins at home, and thrifty girls could not agree more! Here is a step-by-step guide on how to give yourself the perfect facial—at home.

Whether you go it solo or have a thrifty girl's beauty night in with some of your beauty buddies, the point is to have fun and get beauty busy.

On a night (or afternoon, when you have evening plans), give yourself the personal gift of pampering. Start by setting the mood with music. Spas like to play new age or classical music in the background. Light a few candles. Pour yourself a glass of wine in a nice stemmed glass or brew a cup of relaxing, detoxifying tea. Pour the tea into a dainty teacup and saucer. Put on a nice robe, pull your hair back in a headband, and slip off your shoes. Slippers are an option, but being barefooted has its benefits to the feet and legs.

For your fabulous at-home facial, you will need:

- cleanser
- exfoliator
- toner
- cotton pads
- 2 tablespoons of Swiss Kris (available at health food stores)
- pot of boiling water
- towel
- 2 to 3 washcloths
- massage cream, or a moisturizer with 2 pumps of skin serum, or a bit of olive oil
- eye cream
- facial mask

To prepare your spa-at-home area beforehand, put your products on a tray so all you have to do is lather and slather yourself to new beauty heights—without searching for this or looking for that. Let the beauty begin:

1. Cleanse the skin with a mild cleanser. Remove gently with a warm-water washcloth.

2. Apply a facial exfoliator to face and neck using gentle circular motions; remove with a warm-water washcloth.

3. Tone the skin with a gentle toner. Apply to the skin with a cotton pad.

4. The next is steaming your face with herbs (the two tablespoons of Swiss Kris). Swiss Kris is actually formulated as a natural laxative. The product is made with lots of skin-loving herbs and is excellent as a facial steaming product. Boil a pot of water on the stove. Turn off. After two minutes, put the Swiss Kris into the water. Allow to steep, uncovered, for five minutes. Put a towel over the head to allow for the most steaming of the face. Put your face over the steam for three to five minutes, turning the head from side to side, allowing the steam to reach all of the facial pores.

5. Take a warm-water washcloth and gently rinse the skin. Allow to dry.

6. Apply a massage-type cream or moisturizing-type cream with a couple of pumps of skin serum, or olive oil. Believe it or not, olive oil is full of skin-loving ingredients, and when massaged, it is completely absorbed into the skin. Using circular motions with the fingertip pads, massage product into the face, neck, and décolleté for at least five to seven minutes.

7. Remove with a washcloth soaked in warm water.

8. Apply a facial mask that is designed for your skin condition. Follow instructions for applying and removing. While mask is working, relax, lie down, and let the music move you.

9. Remove the mask with a washcloth soaked in warm water.

10. Apply toner to a cotton pad and go over face, neck, and décolleté.

11. Finish your beautiful facial with an application of a deep hydrating moisturizer and eye cream.

If you want to, you can pluck your eyebrows or give yourself a manicure or pedicure. The main thing is to schedule time for beauty and yourself—and maybe your beauty friends!

Chapter Nine

Eyebrow Wow

" There are women who know how to do their makeup perfectly, their hair is always in the latest style, and their choice in fashion is both chic and unique—but their eyebrows just ruin the look. "

—KEVYN AUCOIN

Ask any makeup artist what is one tool you should never leave home without, and the answer will always be a good pair of tweezers. The professionals know that perfectly shaped eyebrows are more flattering than any cosmetic product that could ever be applied. Correctly shaped and colored eyebrows make the eyes appear larger and the face appear slimmer and shapely, accentuate and frame the eyes, and minimize any facial flaws. The right brow will allow the wearer to look stylish and well groomed, no matter what she is wearing. And all this for as little as the cost of tweezers or wax! Great-shaped brows can even mimic an eyelift—without the surgery!

Eyebrows express our emotions best. Pretend for a moment that you are surprised, angry, worried, and suspicious. Without a doubt, each and every time your brows changed to reflect the emotion. Do you remember the famous picture of Vivian Leigh, in the role of Scarlett O'Hara, posed on the steps of Tara, expressionless except for one raised eyebrow? With that one raised eyebrow, Scarlett spoke volumes.

The right brows can be an incredible beauty asset, while the wrong ones can spoil the look of an otherwise pretty face. In fact, changing the brow shape can change the way others perceive you, giving a more sexy, smart, or confident look—without even changing your hairstyle or switching lipsticks!

There has been an emphasis on brows ever since moviegoers saw what a brow could do for a face in the silent movies of yesteryear. The popularity of brows and their grooming continually catches the beauty media industry's eye with articles on places to go for the best brows, and whose brow is hot and whose is not.

Raising the perfect eyebrow is not as hard as it may look. A few simple tricks of the trade are all that is necessary to create your perfect eyebrow wow!

BROW BEAT

If "wild and wooly" describes the look of your brow hair, try a brow setting product. Brow set comes in a mascara type of tube, complete with a mascara brush wand. The difference is that the contents are either clear or creamy and turn to clear when set. To apply, color your brows as usual. Comb them gently into place and brush your brows with the brow set, following the shape of your brows. Once it dries, wild hairs are a thing of the past. Brow setting products are like mousse for your brows.

If do-it-yourself is your plan of action, begin with a pair of flat-slant tweezers. The slant version is the easiest to control. Using natural light, such as light from your bathroom or bedroom window, look into a magnifying mirror to see any stray hairs and begin tweezing—one hair at a time. Go slowly, seeking out each stray hair. Single hair removal is best as it allows you to control the brow shape and not overtweeze.

Before tweezing, first comb the brow hair upwards to see how your hair grows. Trim the brow hair across the very top of the brow hair growth; this will allow your natural brow shape to emerge.

THE BEST TIMES TO TWEEZE

It is best not to tweeze when you are overly tired or stressed. If you do, you will have a tendency to overpluck as you take out your frustrations. Remember the famous reality rule—overpluck, you are stuck!

If tweezing is painful, try taking ibuprofen at least one half hour before tweezing. This will help decrease swelling and inflammation.

The best time to tweeze is after your shower, as the hot water from the shower will open up the pores, and allow for smoother and less painful tweezing.

The worst time to tweeze, or wax, is right before your period. The skin is the most sensitive at this time.

If you are particularly sensitive, try putting your tweezers in the freezer for about thirty minutes before tweezing. The cold has a mild numbing effect on the skin, so it will hurt less.

If waxing is your method of choice, please avoid if you are using AHAS (alpha hydroxyl acids), vitamin A, retinol, or any acne treatment. These types of treatments make the skin prone to sensitivity. To wax when using these medications may mean pulling off the skin underneath as well. Not pretty by any standards.

Develop the habit of combing your brows into shape by taking a brow brush, or an old toothbrush dedicated to this purpose, and combing brows into place. Brush the brows up and over to put in place. By daily brushing into place, the brows will naturally grow into place.

EYEBROW COLOR

For the most believable brow color, use a universal taupe color in a brow pencil. Taupe is the best color to blend with most individuals' coloring. You can change the color intensity by applying pressure (to make it color darker) or by keeping lighter pressure (in the cases of redheads and blondes). If you prefer a brow powder, try using two colors mixed together for the most natural shade. Most cosmetic companies offer brow products in the range of blondes, brunettes, redheads, and even shades of gray in order to blend with hair coloring.

TINT HINT

Eyebrow (and eyelash) tinting is a great way to wake up with brows. Tinting, using a vegetable dye and done professionally in a spa or salon setting, allows lashes and brows to have color for about four weeks. This method is great for fair-haired gals whose natural brow coloring tends to blend into the skin. Plus, having your brows and lashes already done helps save time in the morning makeup routine. Always be sure that the person is experienced in eyebrow and eyelash dyeing, as these dyes can be blinding if used improperly.

When applying brow color, begin at the outside tail and go toward the center of the eye, then continue feathering the brow color all the way to the beginning of the brow. By starting at the end and feathering the brow color on the skin underneath the brow, you are able to fill in any gaps when brow hair may be sparse. Once you have applied the color, gently brush the brows up and back into place. The brush will help remove any excess color, return the brows to their natural shape, and create a groomed, professional look. Once you have achieved your brow look, very lightly pat a bit of translucent powder over the brows to set.

Chapter Ten

Thirty Thrifty Tips for Glamorous Skin

" In the factory we make cosmetics;
in the store we sell hope. "

—CHARLES REVSON

T his chapter covers thirty tips every thrifty girl should know to achieve glamorous skin, on a budget! The better you take care of your skin on a regular basis, the less money you have to spend constantly trying to make it look healthier.

1. When sleeping, keep the heat in the bedroom at a lower setting. Excess heat can cause puffiness in the face and especially around the eyes.

2. Cleanse your face before working out. Moisturizer and makeup keep the pores from expelling toxins such as sweat. Allow the skin to have a little breathing time. Be sure to cleanse, tone, and hydrate the skin post-exercise.

3. Keep your washcloths, towels, and pillowcases free of fabric softener when doing the laundry. Some of the ingredients in fabric softeners are designed to coat the fabric to make it soft. Unfortunately, these coating ingredients are one of the major culprits of sudden breakouts.

4. When cleansing the skin, put your hair back in a headband. With the hair pulled back, you can deep-clean all parts of the face thoroughly—not just dab underneath the bangs or sides of hair.

5. If your skin has a tendency to be puffy, cut down on your salt intake, including sodas. Salt retains water, and usually that excess water is noticed on the face, hands, and ankles.

6. To make the most of your facial mask, heat a damp towel in the microwave for ten to fifteen seconds; apply on top of the mask, and relax as the mask penetrates even better than it would without. You can also use the damp towel to help remove the product more easily.

7. If you are plagued with blackheads and don't have time for a full facial, try one of the pore-cleansing strips that remove blackheads. Be sure to cleanse the skin afterwards and apply a toner to keep the area clean and bacteria-free.

8. Carry a tiny container of moisturizer in your bag. If your skin starts to feel dry during the day, dab on a small amount, especially around the eyes and sides of the lips.

9. Keep a tube of lip moisturizer on your nightstand. Lips do not have any oil glands and are prone to drying out as you sleep, especially if you sleep with your mouth open. The moment you turn out the light, turn on the lip conditioner.

10. Calm down irritated skin with green tea. Brew a tea bag in a teacup for a minimum of five minutes. Pour the tea into a washcloth, squeeze out the excess, and place the cloth over the entire face, pressing the cloth onto the contours of the face. Relax for ten minutes. If the skin still feels irritated, resoak the cloth and repeat.

11. Keep all of your skin care products in one place. A wicker or plastic basket is perfect to store all of your glamour goods, making it easier to have beauty right at your fingertips.

12. If you are prone to breakouts during times of stress, try taking a couple of antacid tablets for a night or two. Excess acid in the system caused from added stress is typically the problem. The antacid tablets will absorb some of the acid, reducing the likelihood of a breakout.

13. Evening primrose oil and vitamin E are two of the most powerful skin supplements available. To increase their benefit even further, take the supplements before going to bed instead of in the morning with your other vitamins. Since the body does most of its repair work while you sleep, taking these two skin-nourishing supplements at night will increase their value, giving you more beautiful skin.

14. Plain yogurt is an excellent facial mask. First, cleanse the skin, and apply contents to face, neck, and décolleté. Relax for fifteen minutes, then remove with a warm-water washcloth. Yogurt contains lactic acid, which works as a natural exfoliator, while the milk proteins gently moisturize the skin.

15. Invest in a mirror that magnifies by three or five times for your grooming area. If possible, choose one with suction cups on the back so you can stick it right on your bathroom mirror. The magnifying mirror will help you prevent makeup smears and streaks by allowing you to see yourself up close and personal—to say nothing about being able to pluck the out-of-thin-air hair that suddenly appears.

16. Treat yourself to a facial smoothie. Place ¼ cup melon, ¼ cup fresh pineapple, and ½ cup of seltzer (or club soda) in a blender. Mix well. Apply to face and neck and relax for fifteen minutes. Rinse with cool water. The pineapple contains enzymes, aiding in dead skin removal. The melon moisturizes, while the seltzer adds a little effervescence to help speed the action of the fruit combo.

17. Start the day with a quick and effective body detox drink. Squeeze the juice of ½ lemon or lime into a mug. Add hot water and drink slowly. This daily ritual will help flush out all the impurities that your body has managed to pick up overnight and prepare your skin for a new day.

18. Start a facial fund. Even if you cannot go for a professional facial as much as you would like, try to schedule at least two a year—one at the end of winter and one at the end of summer. When the season changes as dramatically as winter and summer, the skin goes through a lot of changes as well. A good, professional facial will remove the "season" from your face, as professional products and techniques can go deeper and penetrate more. You will love the results!

19. Sunglasses are all the fashion rage—plus these glamorous accessories are also anti-agers for the eyes. Sunglasses protect the eyes from wrinkling due to the harmful UVA and UVB sunrays. In addition to lessening wrinkles, sunglasses help protect the eyes from overexposure to the sunlight, which can cause inflammation of the cornea and even cataracts. To keep the eyes cooler in warmer climates, look for sunglass lenses with infrared protection.

20. Extra absorbent cotton pads and balls soak up liquids, like toner, all too quickly. Dampen the cotton with water first and squeeze out the excess before putting the toner on the cotton. You will use less product. This tip is also excellent for sensitive skins, since toning products can sometimes tingle.

21. Don't forget to put your sunscreen on the back of the neck, at the hairline, and especially on the ears. These areas are often forgotten—until it's too late.

22. To seal an extra bit of moisture on the skin, try spritzing the face with mineral water after cleansing and toning the skin just before you put on your moisturizer. This will plump up the skin and lock in the moisture for up to 12 hours.

23. To get the most from skin care treatment products, rub them in your hands before applying. This will produce a warming effect and make the product easier to spread.

24. When cleansing, toning, and moisturizing the skin, use upward, circular motions. Gravity is constantly pulling the skin down, so fight back by going up. Using upward motions also stimulates circulation, allowing the products to work better.

25. Sunscreen's active ingredients typically have a two-year shelf life. Write the date you purchase the product on the bottle itself, and toss it out after two years. If it changes color, separates, or has an odd odor before then, be safe and throw it out. You only have one skin.

26. When trying a new product for the first time, it is better to try it at night. In case your skin does not agree with the new product, your skin has several hours to calm down.

27. Keep skin care products out of sunlight. Direct sunlight can cause the product to change consistency or turn bad. Also keep sunscreen products out of the sun. Keep them under the blanket or in your bag.

28. In warm weather, keep your skin care products in the refrigerator. The chill can revive an overly hot face in no time. This is a great tip for days when you have to come home from a hard day's work and be glamorous in the evening.

29. Save the soap for the body—not the face. The best way to cleanse the face is with a liquid or gel facial cleanser. Soap, even soap designed for facial use, contains ingredients that are too harsh for the skin. Think about it—what is exactly keeping the bar a bar?

30. Radiant skin requires a healthy diet, lots of water, exercise, and plenty of rest. Smoking, excess sun exposure, and too much alcohol are menaces to the skin, causing lines and wrinkles and discoloration. All the cleansers, creams, peels, and even face-lifts in the world don't mean a thing, if you are not living a healthy lifestyle. Good health is very glamorous.

PART 3

THE
THRIFTY
GIRL'S
GUIDE TO
GLAMOROUS
MAKEUP

A Thrifty Girl always looks her best—whether running errands or running an important meeting. This section will give advice on the best ways to make yourself up on a budget—no matter what the occasion.

Chapter Eleven

Makeup Matters

" You would be surprised how much
it costs to look this cheap! "
—DOLLY PARTON

Have you ever seen those revealing photographs of models and celebrities caught without any makeup on? While the paparazzi can certainly overstep their boundaries, let's face it: it does give a certain amount of satisfaction to all of us that even the beautiful people look exactly like us sans makeup. Seeing the likes of Gwyneth, Jessica, and Ashley looking like the "befores" proves what Cindy Crawford said is true: "Even I don't wake up looking like Cindy Crawford!"

This chapter is all about products and techniques that you can use to take your face from your own "before" to your very glamorous "after." Stars know it. Makeup artists do it. And now you, too, will be able to create a face worthy of any red carpet—and without spending a fortune!

LAYING THE RIGHT FOUNDATION

The importance of foundation cannot be underestimated. As the first product that touches the skin after moisturizer, it is the "foundation" of a perfect makeup application. There are five types of foundation, all with unique benefits.

Liquid

Liquid foundations are the most versatile, as they work for a full range of skin types. Liquids blend easily, and offer various degrees of coverage. Some formulas even feature moisturizers for drier skin and sunscreens for added protection. The majority of liquid foundations are water based, although some cosmetic lines geared for the mature, drier-skinned clients will have an oil-based foundation.

Cream

Cream foundations are best known for a heavier coverage and added moisturizers. Extra-dry, dry, and normal skin are best suited for cream foundations. Since the base of cream foundation is often oil, combination and oily skin will feel that the consistency is too rich.

Wet/Dry

Compact foundations that can be used either wet for a more sheer finish, or used dry for more coverage, are ideal as they travel well. All skin types can use a compact foundation; it is a matter of choice.

Stick

Stick foundation has come a long way since the days of "movie makeup." Once it was made extremely thick to hold up under studio lights, but now technology has been able to keep the coverage without the pancake feel and look.

Tinted Moisturizer

Tinted moisturizer foundations are great ways to combine steps as the moisturizer is built into the color. Tinted moisturizers give the sheerest of all coverage and are good for oily skin, or skin needing very little coverage.

THE FINISHING TOUCH

Which finish is for you? Dewy or matte? Although a finish is usually used in terms of marketing, any skin can wear either finish. It is a matter of personal preference.

Matte

Matte finishes are good for combination and oily skin types, if only for dulling the natural shine that these skin conditions produce. Matte finish is also the perfect choice for photographs and events where you cannot touch up.

Dewy

Dewy finish foundation just adds a little glisten to the skin. Dry, normal, and especially extra-dry skin types love the look of a dewy finish as it gives the impression of a more moist skin.

Once you have decided upon the type and finish of your foundation, you have to choose the perfect color for your skin.

YOUR PERFECT COLOR

Foundation is like priming the canvas for a painting. You get your color from blush, eye shadow, and lip color. Foundation should simply blend into your natural skin tone.

A foundation's job is to create the most flawless look possible for your skin. It should blend away blemishes and discolorations. Choosing a color that is the closest match possible to your skin tone will make you appear younger, more polished, and, believe it or not—smarter!

CLEAN AND FRESH

Keep your makeup area clean. Toss all your half-used, held-together-with-a-rubber-band containers and nubs of eye and lip pencils. How can you feel "glamorous" when you are applying "downtrodden" products? You would not think of eating old, dirty food, so keep it fresh on the face as well.

In order to choose the perfect tone of foundation, it is necessary to see the color against your skin in natural lighting. While most stores have fluorescent and other types of light, natural lighting is what will determine your shade. If you are trying foundations in anything but natural lighting, take a hand mirror and go to the nearest window to see up close what the color truly looks like against your skin.

The best way to test foundation is to apply a small amount directly on the jawline. If it is the right color, the foundation will disappear from view, leaving only skin that looks smoother and more flawless.

NOW ACCEPTING APPLICATIONS

Now that you have the formula and the color, it is time to apply. Begin by dotting the face with five dots of foundation: one on the forehead, one on each cheek, one on the nose, and one on the chin. Using a sponge, a foundation brush, or clean fingers, begin blending the foundation evenly over the skin's surface using long sweeping strokes. Be sure to blend the foundation into the hairline and smooth out areas around the nose and eyes. To ensure that any little facial hair lies down, take a sponge and gently go downward to the jawline to finish.

DO YOU HAVE ANYTHING TO CONCEAL?

Concealers can cover a multitude of sins—from dark under-eye circles to blemishes that appear overnight to scars and discolorations. Choosing the right formula is like choosing a foundation. Formulas come in stick, pot, wet or dry, and liquid. While again it is a personal preference, one of the most versatile formulas is in the pot. A pot formula is a little thicker, allowing for better staying power and less straying as your face warms up.

Concealers are best applied before the foundation. This allows the concealer to directly cover the situation, and by smoothing foundation over the concealer, it gives a more flawless look—avoiding raccoon eyes or spotlights where a blemish is covered.

To apply, use the ring finger and gently pat the product onto the skin. Allow the product to warm up before applying it to sensitive places such as the tender under-eye area. Pat the product until it feels slightly dry, which means it is setting. Wait one to two minutes before applying foundation to ensure that the concealer is set. Here are some inexpensive concealers to try:

- Skin Pearls
- Physician's Formula

TAKE A POWDER

Once the concealer and foundation are in place, it is time to set it with a light dusting of powder. Powder does for the face what hair spray does for the hair—it sets it and keeps your handiwork looking great from sunrise to sunset.

Powder has come a long way in the last few years. Now most formulas are very finely milled, allowing for more than one application of powder without looking cakey. Before, dry skin types dreaded applying powder as it usually emphasized wrinkles and crinkles instead of hiding them like the new types of powders do. Some formulas even contain light diffusing ingredients to make the skin appear younger and more radiant. Try these brands:

- Hard Candy Complexion Perfections
- Models Prefer

Using a large powder brush, gently go all over the face with a dusting of powder. The powder can be loose or compact, whichever you prefer. The larger the powder brush, the fewer mistakes you can make with powder. Simply glide the brush along from the top of the face to the jawline. Plus, there is something downright glamorous about a big, fluffy powder brush. It just feels glamorous as you see the powder brush gliding across your face.

YOU'RE BLUSHING

Blusher is one of the hardest cosmetics to apply. It must be blended perfectly so there is no start or stop to the color. In addition, blush, when properly applied, brings out your best facial features, such as great cheekbones, beautiful eyes, luscious lips, or perfect chin. The right color of blush will give you a healthy glow—the wrong blush color will make you look tired, drained, and overdone.

Like our other color cosmetics, blush must be chosen to reflect the right color for you. Matching your blusher to your lip color or clothes is an outdated method. Choose instead to find a blusher that looks good on you—no matter what you are wearing. A good rule of *thumb* is to use your thumb when selecting colors. Your thumb color is, by far, the very best natural blush color for you. Simply select blush colors by comparing the colors to the color of your thumb. Blush should look like you have color in your cheeks naturally—the color you would be if you had done a few minutes of exercise.

Apply blush to the face after your foundation and powder, unless you are using a cream blush. Cream blushes should go on the skin after foundation, but before powder.

When using a powder blush, apply it after your powder. Remember to powder the skin again, after applying blush, to set the blush to withstand the usual afternoon makeup meltdown syndrome.

For the most natural-looking blush application, start by putting the blush on the cheekbones, halfway between the top and the bottom of the ear. Sweep the blush upward toward the temple and hairline, almost like the shape of a comma. Keeping the blush above the imaginary line where the nose ends, and stopping where the center of the iris is in the eye will give the most flattering contour to the cheeks. Blush, when properly applied, is like a face-lift, drawing the eye upward toward your beautiful eyes.

Blush formulas include powder, cream, liquid or gel, and pencils. Each has its own benefits.

Powder Blush

This is by far the easiest and most versatile to use. Perfect for all skin conditions, powder blush is very sheer and natural looking. Housed in a compact, powder blush is easy to transport, making touch-ups a breeze. Because powder is sheer, it is easy to layer using two or more colors to create accent cheekbones and temples and to slim the sides of the nose.

Cream Blush

This is a great way to blush for normal to dry skin. Cream blush offers more intense color than powder, so use sparingly and blend well. Cream blush contains more moisturizers than powders, so they cling better and tend to last longer on extra-dry, dry, and normal skin.

Liquid or Gel Blush

Liquid and gels last the longest on the skin, as they are usually oil-free and produce a translucent "stain" on the skin. This type of blush takes practice, as once you apply the color you have a very short window of opportunity to spread it before the stainlike effect is in place. One benefit to liquid and gels is that most formulas are water-resistant enough to even swim in. To apply this type of blush, start with a very small amount, quickly spread into place, and if more color is needed, add another bit—gradual is the key to a natural look.

PIGGYBACKING BLUSH

To make your blush industrial strength, after applying foundation, apply cream blush, powder as usual, and then apply a powder blush to the skin. This is called "piggybacking" the product onto the skin. Makeup artists use this technique all the time when they need a look to last all day.

Be sure to apply another layer of powder to the face after applying this method, as the powder is what sets the face and allows the finished look to last well into the night!

Blush Pencils or Sticks

Blush pencils and sticks are easy to apply, as the color goes right where you put it. Blush pencils and sticks can be either creamy or in the form of a gel. To apply, stroke the pencil or stick upward on the cheeks. Using the finger, or a sponge, gently blend in the color so there is no edge to where the blush starts or stops.

Bronzers

Want a sun-kissed look, no matter what the season? Bronzing products are a quick way to put the tropics into your cheeks or all over the face. Bronzers require some practice to be able to create that subtle glow and not make it look like your skin is dirty. Bronzers come in powder, liquid, and gels. The easiest way to learn the art of bronzing is to start with a powder bronzer and a large powder brush. Gently glide the powder brush across the powder and apply to the areas of the face where the sun would naturally hit—like across the cheeks and nose. Once you have mastered that technique, you can try your hand at liquids and gels for an all-over sun goddess look. Remember, less is more. It is so much easier to apply more product than it is to have to take it off and start over!

THRIFTY TIP

Nothing ages you faster than out-of-date makeup. If you have not updated your look in the last five years, it shows! Make an appointment with your favorite cosmetic company and ask for a free makeover. All companies offer complimentary consultations. Some even offer makeup lessons to teach you how to bring out your very best features. It may only take an adjustment or two to keep you current.

While the sky is the limit on how much these products can cost, Thrifty Girls know that sometimes you need to splurge on some and save on others. To get the biggest bang for your buck, plan on spending a little more for your foundation. Foundation is the first product that is applied directly to the skin. Choosing a formula that is good for your skin and matches properly is a grand investment. You will look more radiant with fewer imperfections. All of the other color products can easily be beauty bargains, but spend a little more for the perfect base. When you see your glamour girl skin in the mirror, you'll be glad you did.

Chapter Twelve

Custom Eyes

" The eyes have no real limitations. Each shape you create, whether with shadows, pencils or liner, can take you into completely different realms. **"**

—KEVYN AUCOIN

W ithout a doubt, the eyes have it. Eyes come in all shapes and sizes, and colors that would give a crystal prism a run for the money. It has been said that eyes are the windows of the soul, as more than 80 percent of the information that is received from the world comes through the eyes. The eyes also tell the world several things about you— your feelings, your state of health, and your age. Eyes are the most expressive feature that you have when you communicate. Eyes can show a complete range of emotions, depending on the setting—from the boardroom to the ballroom.

Learning to emphasize, and customize, your eyes to their best advantage will serve you well in your quest for beauty and glamour. Knowing what techniques to use when you want to project a very glamorous look, and which methods to use for your professional yet elegant workday image, are skills worth their weight in gold shimmer.

GLAMOROUS EYES ON A THRIFTY BUDGET

Buying eye makeup is a thrifty girl's delight, as the products can all be found at reasonable prices—you don't have to spend a lot of money to make your eyes your beauty focal point. Cosmetic companies all are competing for your business, and each one offers a great array of products to choose from.

THRIFTY TIP

When you are choosing eye makeup, especially if you're experimenting, it's best to go to the drugstore instead of the cosmetic counters. There are dozens of quality brands available for reasonable prices. The hardest part is choosing which color to buy!

THE ART OF ILLUSION

There are several products a Thrifty Girl can use to achieve the most glamorous look. Here is some important information on all of these elements.

Eye Shadow

What makeup colors look best on you is primarily determined by your skin tone and what you're wearing. Eye and hair color are the second most important factors to consider. Your clothes closet is a good guide for choosing your eye coloring products. If you wear warm, earth-toned colors, such as olive green, brown, terra-cotta, and camel, warm tones are probably your best bets for eye color. If most of your clothes are in the cool tones of blue, purple, lavender, dark green, and red, cool color will look great on your eyes. Of course, the neutrals of gray, ivory, taupe, and brown are excellent choices for times that you cannot make up your mind, or if you decide to wear black, red, white, or beige clothing.

With the choices of eye shadow colors and textures, no wonder it can look complicated to apply. While makeup artists often go for a fantasy look found on the runway—and *only* the runway—most artists agree that two shades of shadow at a time (one darker and one lighter) are what you need in the runway of life.

BAG LADY

Take all your carry-along makeup items in a clear makeup bag. It keeps your products together in one place, cleanly and neatly. Plus, since the bag is see-through, retouching your powder and lip color is a snap because you know exactly where to find each item. Changing handbags will be a breeze, as you just grab your makeup bag and go.

Don't let the Glamour Girl in you scare the Thrifty Girl. A wardrobe of only three or four colors of eye shadow can take you from day to evening and back again. A sheer light shade is good for the background of the eyes, as this color will sweep on the eyelid from lash line to brow, creating a canvas for the eyes. Natural pink, light peach, or buff are good choices. A second, darker color will add the drama by creating a shadow in the eye crease and corners of the eyes. Gray, brown, and perhaps a smoky purple are excellent choices to start your makeup wardrobe. Pick a trendy color now and then to keep up with the fashion— but only if you think it looks good on your eyes. Somehow the reds and neon shades never quite look as if they belong on anyone older than fourteen, and they end up sitting in the bottom of your makeup case—talk about a waste of a beauty budget!

Here are a few brands to try:

- Too Faced
- L'oreal

Eye shadows come in three different forms: creams, pencils, and powders.

> **CREAMS** are the hardest to control as they contain ingredients that keep them soft in the container. Unfortunately, those ingredients can also make the shadow slip and crease on the eyelid.

> **PENCILS** are easy to use—simply swipe and blend on the lid. Some pencils can also slip and slide if the formula is too moisturizing.

> **POWDERS** provide the longest-lasting eye shadow wear. Powder can be used wet or dry, glides on, is almost mistake-proof, and lasts and lasts. Some of the new moisturizing formulas could be a little *too* moisturizing. A quick

test is to run your finger over the powder lightly. If your finger glides very quickly, it could contain too much moisture for you. If, on the other hand, your finger sticks in place, the formula could be too dry for your eyelids and look cakey after applying. A little moisture is a good thing, as the shadow will cling where it belongs and protect the lids at the same time.

THRIFTY TIP

For goodness' sake, toss the little sponge applicators that come with the eye shadow! They are way too stiff and small to maneuver and do an awful job of blending the shadow. Use an eye shadow brush instead, which is inexpensive and can be found in your drugstore. Brushes allow the product to glide on and blend wonderfully. Plus, a brush will never scrape your skin like the dumb free ones that come with the product.

To create industrial strength–lasting eye shadow wear, try an eye shadow primer before putting the eye shadow on. Shadow primers are taupe, nude, or creamy. They're light in color, and once applied, look like the lid color. Shadow primer contains ingredients that cling to the skin and keep a slight barrier between your lid and the eye shadow color, keep body oils away from the shadow, and allow for longer wear without smearing and creasing in the crease of the eyelid.

Eyeliner

Eyeliner adds the pizzazz to eye makeup. By outlining the eyes, eyeliner frames and defines the eyes, drawing attention to them. Eyeliners come in pencils, cakes, powders, and liquid.

Liquid, by far, is the hardest method to master. It is best saved for the experts or when you have plenty of time to start over, if need be! Pencils, cakes, and powders are much more user-friendly and forgiving. Pencils can be made of powder or crayon-type consistency.

Use eyeliner pencils as you would a regular pencil. Hold with your fingers near the point and gently apply a line across the eyes, near both the upper and lower lashes.

Cakes and powders come in a pot and are applied with either a pointed brush or a flat-sided brush. A flat-sided brush allows the product to be placed right where the brush goes. To add more, simply reload the brush and place on the next area. Pointed eyeliner brushes glide along the lids to create the line like a paintbrush.

> ## BLEND, BLEND, BLEND
> No matter the product, remember to blend. Have a supply of cotton swabs on hand to smooth any harsh start and stop lines. Liners should create drama, yet allow the eyes to be the stars. People should notice your beautiful eyes—not your eye makeup.

Colors used to line the eyes should be subtle and determined by your choice for eye shadow colors. Good basics are brown, gray, and navy for most looks. Unless you have dark hair and eyes, black liner can be overpowering. While it worked for Cleopatra, it could be a little much for you. To add a little zip to your makeup routine, add a trendy color now and then for fun—like a smoky purple or teal. Try these inexpensive brands:

- Bourjois Khol & Contour Eyeliner
- Prestige Eye Pencil

Mascara

The perfecting finishing to beautiful eyes is mascara. Mascara darkens and thickens the eyelashes and makes them appear longer. Mascara comes in cake and wand. Cake is a bit trickier to use, as it requires getting used to. The cake is dry, and you need to add water (never saliva) to the cake make a creamy paste to apply. Cake mascara was the first type of mascara and has been around since the days of silent films. While it may not be practical to use on a daily basis, there is something very Hollywood about it. The wand is the perennial favorite, both for ease of use and because the wand brushes will help curl the lashes as the mascara is applied.

Standard colors of mascara are brown, black/brown, and black. Black mascara is the color that most women (and makeup artist) prefer, and for good reason. Black mascara is the little black dress for the eyes—it looks great on just about everyone. But if you are really light blonde or a redhead, brown is probably a more suitable choice. Otherwise—make it black!

Mascara can be water-resistant or waterproof. Water-resistant is a better choice, as waterproof is hard on the eyelashes. When it dries, it contracts, causing stress to be placed on the lashes, and can actually cause them to break or fall out before their time. Besides, waterproof will smear if you touch it while crying or swimming—so why stress out your lashes? Go with the water-resistant.

Mascara formulas can contain lengthening fibers, curling agents, and thickeners. Lengthening fibers will add tiny mascara colored fibers that will cling to the lashes, giving the illusion of longer lashes. Curling mascara contains ingredients that actually cause the eyelashes to curl a bit. Thickening formulas will create depth, making the lashes look thicker and richer with color.

Plan on keeping your mascara for only about three to four months, tops, as mascara can harbor bacteria. Pumping the wand with the brush is not a good idea. This causes the formula to dry out faster due to the amount of air being pushed into the tube with the pumping action. Instead, close the container and reopen to reload the brush. Either way, it needs the boot after three to four months. I recommend these reasonably priced brands:

- Bourjois Volume Glamour Mascara
- Maybelline Great Lash

To apply, start at the lower lashes and lightly brush a coat of mascara on the lashes. On the top, start with the outside of the lashes and work inward, using small zigzag like movements to apply. Zigzagging will both color and separate the lashes at the same time, allowing for less clumping and better color coverage. To have one coat of mascara do the work of two, put the mascara brush on the top of the lashes and roll outward. This colors the top of the lashes, making them appear fuller. For daytime, one coat is usually fine, especially if you choose a thickening formula. For evenings out, a second coat will create the glamour girl look.

If using an eyelash curler, be sure to curl the lashes *before* applying mascara, as curling with mascara on causes the lashes to break. To create the most curl to the lash, start by putting the lash curler on the base of the lashes near the lid skin. Crimp the curler. Count to twenty and then release. To add even more curl, continue by putting the lash curler halfway down the lash and curl for additional count to ten. This will give the lashes double-duty curling action that lasts all day.

LOOKING AT EYE SHAPES

The key to the art of eye makeup application is being able to successfully create illusions. Any "faults" you perceive about your eyes—wide-set, close-set, small, large, too much lid, deep-set, or the like—can be easily be made to be more beautiful, youthful, bright and expressive with a stroke of this shadow, a dab of that liner, and a whisk or two of volumizing mascara. It is all in the know-how.

FISHING FOR COMPLIMENTS

Do as the pros do and keep your makeup organized in a fishing tackle box. It comes with a carrying handle, top and bottom compartments, and loads of little areas to stash makeup extras and keep all of your colors together. Plastic is lighter than metal and is easy to wipe down if something spills.

Highlighting and shading are the two basic techniques used to enhance the eye's natural shape. The most effective colors to combine with this technique are matte, neutral shades. Remember, neutral is not limited to brown and gray; in fact, neutral just means soft colors found in skin. Colors like beige, vanilla, mauve, and, yes, brown and gray. But neutrals also include gold, olive, pale purple, and even shades of blue. Neutrals are easy to work with because the colors meld well with one another as well as compliment the skin tone.

THRIFTY TIP

Sometimes you can find an array of eyeshadow colors all in one palette, which will provide variety for less money.

To make your eyes look a certain way, follow these tips:

CLOSER TOGETHER: Apply a light or medium neutral shade of eye shadow on the inner corner of the eyelid. Add eyeliner to draw a line that is slightly thicker on the inner corners of the eye and thin the liner line out as you go toward the outside corner where the eye ends.

FARTHER APART: Apply a matte colored shadow in a slightly darker shade than your regular shadow; sweep it outward and slightly upward on the outer corners of the top and bottom lids. Add eyeliner. Starting slightly past where the eye begins, allow the liner line to thicken upon extending to the outside part of the eye, tilting the liner up toward the end.

LARGER: If you want your eyes to look larger, add lightness to them. As light tones enlarge, and darker tones recede, the trick to bigger eyes is to add some light. Apply light neutral eye shadow color in the crease of your lid above the iris. If you want a bit more color, add the color on the lid, but keep the lighter color slightly peeking above. The light behind the lid color acts like a sunset over the ocean. Another way to increase the illusion of larger eyes is to apply a neutral color on the entire eye lid and then a contour (darker) color in the eye's crease and along the outer upper and lower outside crease. Add eyeliner by following the natural shape of the eye along the top and bottom of the eyelashes.

ROUNDER: Apply eye shadow all around the edges of the upper and lower lids. Add eyeliner to outline the eye at the base of the lashes. As you move the eyeliner toward the outside of the eye, slightly thicken the liner and "wing" it upward, à la Brigitte Bardot.

PERFECTLY OVAL: Apply eye shadow over the entire eyelid, from lashes to brow. Add a contour (darker) shadow in the shape of a C from the outside corner inward in the crease, and add a slight smudge of color on the outside corner. Add eyeliner right at the base of the lashes. Thicken it slightly in the middle of the lid, and draw it toward the outer corner.

Chapter Thirteen
Lip Appeal

" Hand me my purse, will you, darling? A girl can't read that sort of thing without her lipstick. "

—AUDREY HEPBURN AS HOLLY GOLIGHTLY IN *BREAKFAST AT TIFFANY'S*

L ip color adds the finishing touch to a look by defining the mouth and adding color to the face. It is also the step during which you can have the most fun, as there are fewer makeup "how-to's" and "no-no's" than anywhere else. You can transform your look simply by changing your lip color. Faster than you can blow a kiss, you can go from the girl next door to the ooh la la glam girl of the moment just by swiping on a different shade of lipstick.

BRAVE HEART

If you have been brave enough to buy a very different color of lip color than what you are used to wearing, try experimenting with the new color over the weekend. Apply the lip color and look at yourself in the mirror every now and then. By allowing yourself the weekend to become used to your new color look, you will gradually train your eye to like it.

Lips are the pivotal point of the face. A great lip color can bring light and focus to a woman's facial features and highlight her smile. It really doesn't matter if the lips are well defined with lipstick and liner, or just dabbed with a bit of gloss—wearing color on the lips is the fastest way to add a little beauty to your looks.

DECISIONS, DECISIONS

Most women have the luxury of owning a variety of lip colors, and of being able to select a particular color that suits the occasion. In fact, studies show that 97 percent of women between ages twenty and forty-five wear lipstick. The study also shows that at least 65 percent of us own more than ten shades!

Your choice of color usually depends on several factors. By taking the following factors into consideration, you can avoid wasting money by buying lipstick that ends up looking terrible on you.

Skin Tone

First, you have to determine whether you have a cool or warm skin tone, and what tone is your skin complexion.

Fair Skin

Fair complexions should seek out mauve browns with complexion-warming pink or peach undertones, depending on cool or warm coloring. For more dramatic color, try a blue-based or cherry-color red with a hint of brown. Women with really pale skin and very dark hair (like Audrey Hepburn and Paloma Picasso) have the luxury to try many colors—especially those with lots of contrast, like fuchsia, bright true red, and even shades of bright coral.

Olive Skin

Thrifty Girls with olive skin look good in light brown or raisin shades, with warm undertones that will light up the face. For a deeper color, browner reds like blackberry or wine are beautiful on olive skin tones.

Dark Skin

Dark skins can carry off the deepest reds of all—those with dark blue or purplish undertones. Deep browns with wine, purple, or bluish tones can look stunning as well.

Don't worry that you cannot wear a certain color. Almost every color has a cool and a warm hue. Think of red—there is valentine red, which is cool, and there is tomato red, which is warm. Shades that look suedelike tend to be more neutral than clear colors.

Clothing Color

Secondly, you should consider what clothing you will be wearing. Lip color should not clash with the color of clothing you are wearing—rather, it should compliment it. If you are wearing a smart red dress, an application of equally balanced red lip color can be highly effective and communicate your confidence.

Style of Dress

Lastly, you need to factor in the style of clothing that you will be wearing. Is your outfit casual wear like jeans and a sweater, a business or luncheon outfit, or is it an evening-out affair? With casual clothing, lip colors on the more natural side go with the look. Business or luncheons need a lip color that is professional—more middle of the road. For evenings out, strong, dark, and full lip colors are the quickest way to chic.

MORE THAN JUST LIPSTICK

Can you remember when lipstick was just lipstick? Today lip colors come in so many different formulations—matte, shiny, glossy, sheer, creamy, long-lasting, and even lip-plumping. Finding the one you want is harder than ever. But if you know what look you are going for—barely there color to full-on glamour—there is a formula for you.

> **MATTE:** Colors are extremely opaque, flat, and very highly pigmented. Matte lip colors offer a maximum amount of wear and can leave a temporary stain on the lips when they wear off, allowing the lips to still look colored.

LONG-LASTING: Long-lasting lip colors are designed to allow you to put color on and have it stay on until you yourself—not wear and tear—take it off. Kiss-proof is the selling point. This formula is the most drying one to the lips. While great advances are being made with this kind of lip color, it takes a special wearer to like the texture and feel of the finished product.

SHINY AND GLOSSY: Colors are very sheer and shiny. This formula has added moisturizing ingredients that can help dry lips. It can be worn alone or with a lip pencil, or you can add shiny/glossy lip colors on top of other formulas to alter the texture and add a bit of shine.

SHEER: This feels ultra-light on the lips and can contain a little shine. Sheer formulas are rich with moisturizers and will wear longer than glossy/shiny formulas. Since this is a summertime favorite, a lot of the sheer colors will have an SPF added to help protect the lips.

CREAMY: Creamy lipsticks provide opaque coverage and can add a little bit of a shine to the look. Creamy formulas contain conditioners and moisturizers so that lips feel smooth, and the color usually wears evenly. Creams are the most popular and thus offer the widest choice of shades.

LIP LINERS

Lip liners are the secret weapon to perfect-looking lips. Used correctly, it will make your lips camera close-up ready. Use it wrongly, and you could be confused for Mommy Dearest.

Makeup artists would not think of "doing the lips" without a lip liner to put the look together. However, lip liners can be intimidating for many women. We've all seen too many cases where the lip liner looked unnatural—drawn on, or a night-and-day different shade from the lip color. No wonder it is the most often skipped step—we don't want to be yet another victim of lip liner blunders. But today's liners are much more useable and believable than liners of the past. The formulas go from matte to creamy, and even to pearlized. They blend beautifully with natural skin tones and lip texture. Lip liners are available in pencil, crayon, and felt-tip pens.

Line Me Up

For the most modern look, sharpen the pencil and then lightly rub the tip over a tissue to soften the tip just a bit. Line the lips where the lip skin meets the facial skin. The best look is to match your lip color to your lip liner, choose a color closely matching your skin tone, or use slightly peachy colored lip liner similar to the color of your lips. That way, if your lip color fades, you will be left without an obvious lip outline.

LIP STABILIZER

Lip stabilizer is like foundation for your lips. Stabilizer comes in a pot, squeeze tube, or in a lipstick tube. The color can be nude or clear. Apply stabilizer before applying the lip liner and lip color in order to create the longest lasting lip color. In addition to helping the lip color last longer, the stabilizer will also help protect against lip color feathering outside the lip lines, and it is excellent to keep lip colors true, preventing an orangey look to the lips, resulting from your natural skin oils mixing with the lip color.

EXTRA EXTRAS

With lip color accessories, you can extend your lip color wardrobe even more. Just take your favorite stand-by-me color and add a sweep of gloss to make it shine. Or how about a hint of shimmering gold or silver to add a little extra lux to the lips? You can line the lips with lip liner, color in the lips with the lip liner, and add the lip color on top to create a longer lasting lip color. Mixing colors is a great way to add variety without adding any extra cost. If you love your newly mixed color creation, be sure to remember how you got it for next time!

LIP SHAPES

The good news is that no lip shape is totally perfect; the better news is that all lip shapes can lean a little more toward perfect with just a few simple lip tricks.

> **THIN LIPS:** First, don't even think about drawing a line outside your natural lip line in some *I Love Lucy* attempt to make your lips appear bigger. It will just make you look messy and unnatural. Instead, add a little fullness by wearing light to medium shades of lip colors. Add a little bit of extra color to the center of the mouth, and then blend it outwards. Bright reds, and very dark lip colors with matte finishes, are not your friend, as with

thinner lips, they will make the lips look like they have been slashed—not colored.

FULL LIPS: Darling, you are in such style now. If you got 'em, flaunt 'em. Women are lining up to have injected what you got in nature. But if you feel like your lips arrive before you do when you enter a room, skip the lip liner and wear paler shades of lip color. Gloss needs the toss, as it only accentuates fullness. Matte is a better choice. To draw attention away from the lips, wear only a hint of lip color, and make your eyes the center of attention.

UNEVEN LIPS: If either your top lip is fuller or your lower lip is bigger than your top, know that you are not alone. Over 80 percent of women are in your boat. To help create balance, outline only the outside edge of the top lip and bottom lip only. To apply, simply purse your lips and apply the liner to the outside one-third of the lips, allowing the liner to simply fade away—without a sharp start-stop line.

WIDE LIPS: To draw attention away from the width of the lips, concentrate the lip liner on your lips' cupid bow. This will add height to the lips and take the emphasis off the width. To create more attention to the center of the mouth, dab a little gold or silver gloss onto the center of the lower lip, over your lip color.

TINY LIPS: Lip colors in medium shades will be the most flattering on smaller lips. Try experimenting with different lip texture formulas, to make even the smallest of lips especially glossy, and shiny tints in bright colors. In fact, bright colors are made for you! You have the lips that can carry the brighter shades off beautifully. Save the lip liner to apply after your lip color is on, as it will make the lips appear larger.

DOWNTURNED LIPS: Appling concealer around the outer edges of the lips will help camouflage any downward turn to the lips. Stay away from darker shades of lip color, choosing instead paler shades. Focus the intensity of the color to the center of the mouth and away from the edges. Sheer formulas are great choices for your lips.

CREATING THE MOST GLAMOUROUS LIPS

Creating the greatest looking lips anytime, anyplace, and anywhere is as simple as connecting the dots. All that is required is that you choose your favorite lip color and texture, and a sharp lip liner, and you are ready to go.

1. Apply a lip stabilizer to the lips.

2. With your lip liner, apply two dots, one at the edge of each corner on either side of the upper lip. Then add two more dots—one on each of the twin peaks in the center of the upper lips (the bows).

3. Connect the dots. First, connect the dot on each corner up to the dot on the bow of the lip on the same side. Then, connect the dots on both bows together to completely outline the top lip.

4. Outline, beginning at the middle of the lower lip, lining outward to the corners of the lips, stopping right as you get to the corners.

5. Apply lip color. Blend any visible edges of lip liner lines with the lip color.

6. Admire your work. Add a little gloss or shimmer if needed. Pucker up—you are beautiful.

Most women feel naked without their lip color. They report that lip color is the cosmetics equivalent of shoes or clothes—it is an instant mood-booster and is much more economical. Plus, you don't have to remove anything to try it on! For the price of a latte or two, you can have a new lip color look. Now that's a Thrifty Girl's dream!

Chapter Fourteen

The Thrifty Girl's Guide to a Perfect Makeup Lesson

" "A little powder and a little paint helps you look like what you ain't! "
—SUSIE GALVEZ

Applying your makeup perfectly every time is easy when you follow these fourteen professional makeup application tips. After you master these, you won't need to visit costly makeup consultants or keep trying to snag free makeover after free makeover.

It is important to remember to always apply makeup to a face that has been cleansed, toned, and moisturized.

1. Eye shadow primer. Apply a very small amount to each eyelid. Be sure to cover the entire eyelid from the lash line up to the brow. Primer helps keep the eye shadow on and reduces creasing.

2. Conceal and correct. Apply a tiny bit of concealer and pat underneath your eyes. Patting, before blending, warms the product and allows for better coverage, especially underneath the tender eye area. Using your ring finger, apply under eyes and anywhere that you experience discoloration, spots, blemishes, and/or scars. Blend lightly.

3. Lip treatment. Apply a small amount of lip stabilizer to the lips. Stabilizer will keep the lipstick colors true, as well as aid in keeping lipstick from bleeding.

4. Foundation. Apply five dots of foundation to the face: one on each cheek and on the forehead, chin, and nose. Using a cosmetic sponge, lightly blend the foundation. To keep demarcation lines away, take the side of the sponge and gently blend foundation up to the hairline and then down toward the chin to allow any fine facial hair to lie down.

5. Powder. Lightly dust finishing powder all over the face, using a big powder brush for the best application. A large powder brush distributes the powder evenly and discourages caking and/or building up of excess in any lines.

6. Blush. Apply blush starting near the middle of ear level on the cheek, where the apple of the cheek is located. Be careful to keep the blush out of the area under the nose or past the center of the eye.

7. Powder. Lightly powder all areas where blush was applied. Powdering will set the blush so that it will last longer.

8. Eye shadow. Apply a light base color of eye shadow to the entire lid area, from the lash line up to the brow. Blend well to avoid any start or stop lines of unblended color.

9. Eyeliner. Begin by lining underneath the eyes. Apply the eyeliner underneath the lashes and gently go back and forth using a feathering technique. Repeat on the top lid as close to lashes as possible. Be sure to go from the outside all of the way to where the lashes stop on the lid inside toward the nose. To soften, use a cotton swab to gently smudge the line. Using your eye shadow brush, add a dab of the light base eye shadow color and gently press into the eyeliner to set the liner for the longest lasting application.

10. Contour eye shadow. To create emphasis to your eyes, use a contour (darker) color on your eyelids. Starting at the outside top lid area, lightly apply the contour color to about one third of the lid area, and then trace over the natural eye contour bone. Creating a C from the outside one-third up and over the contour bone area will add definition to the eyes and create a bit of depth.

11. Mascara. Starting with the bottom lashes, gently coat lashes with mascara. Repeat on the top lashes using a zig-zag method of application. Starting at the lash root, take the mascara wand and make small zigzag movements up and out toward the lash tip. Then place the mascara wand on the top of the lashes and roll the wand out, grabbing the tip of the lashes. To finish, zigzag the lashes back up for the most maximum curl. For a really glamorous look, add a second coat.

12. Brow. Apply brow color from the outside of the brow inward toward the brow beginning. Starting at the tail of the brow, begin to color the skin underneath the brow hair with brow color. Continue coloring up and all the way to the beginning of the brow. Tame the look by using a brow comb to gently comb brows back into place.

13. Lip liner. Begin by lining the natural contours of the lips. Then continue by filling in the lip area with lip liner to create the longest lasting lipstick application.

14. Lip color. Apply your favorite lip color and top with gloss if you like.

Smile and say *"Hello, Beautiful!"*—because you are.

If you like, make a copy of this guide and tape it your bathroom mirror or put it on your counter and follow these easy steps until you feel like a Glamour Girl pro!

Chapter Fifteen

Thirty Thrifty Tips for Marvelous Makeup

" Beauty, to me, is about being comfortable in your own skin. That or a kick-ass red lipstick. "

—GWYNETH PALTROW

Here are thirty thrifty tips for Glamour Girls to make themselves up, marvelously!

1. Buy a pretty powder compact or mirror for your purse. While it may cost a little more than a plain one, you will feel so glamorous each and every time you powder your nose or reapply your lipstick.

2. When testing a new lip color, instead of swiping the colors on the back of your hand, use your thumb instead. Thumb and lip color are very close, so you will be able to see how the color will actually look.

3. Keep makeup pencils sharp for a better application. Sharpening pencils also removes any bacteria from the point. But it only takes a quick turn or two with the sharpener—overdoing will waste product.

4. Always dry your hair before applying your makeup. The heat from the dryer can make you perspire and cause your makeup to smudge.

5. Sometimes, just for fun, get together with a girlfriend and do each other's makeup. You will be amazed at how people think you look best, even if you have been lifelong friends. Plus, it is a great way to find a new look.

6. Try moistening foundation with a spritz of oil-free toner on the sponge instead of water. You will get the slip that you need to spread the foundation, and a little extra treatment to boot.

7. To revive powder makeup products that have gotten a little cakey from your skin oils, take a butter knife and gently scrape off the top coating. The powder underneath will once again be fresh and new.

8. Don't remove the entire plastic protection from facial powders. Instead, poke a few holes in it to allow powder to come through. When applying, shake the powder onto the lid and load your brush. You will save lots of powder and don't have to worry about spilling it.

9. Another way to store your facial powder is in a salt shaker. Put some powder in a glass salt shaker. Shake some into your hand and glide your powder brush across, then apply. You can even custom blend two or more colors of powder for the perfect powder color combination for you.

10. Proper makeup application calls for proper lighting. Change the light bulbs in your grooming area to bulbs at least 60 watts, or, if using a lighted makeup mirror, check the wattage to ensure that the bulbs are at least 25 watts each.

11. A lip brush is a glamorous way to apply lip color. Lip color will glide on effortlessly with a back and forth motion. Be sure to choose a lip brush that closes securely. Lip color only looks good on the lips—not on the purse!

12. Exfoliate the lips every month to remove dead skin and oil buildup. You can buy lip exfoliating products, but an easy and thrifty way to new-feeling lips is to apply a coating of petroleum jelly to the lips. Then gently rub a toothbrush (that is used only for this purpose) back and forth. Rinse with warm water, and be sure to put a little lip conditioner on the lips for protection.

13. For dance-proof eye shadow, wet the shadow before applying, but instead of water, use a couple of drops of eyedrops instead. The eyedrops will form a paste with the shadow and allow for a smoother and longer lasting application. Allow to set and you will be all set!

14. Clean cosmetic brushes and applicators in antibacterial soap at least once a month, rinse, put bristles in original brush shape, and let air-dry. Brushes can harbor bacteria and excess makeup.

15. To spotlight your eyes, place a small (about the size of a dime) dot of a golden or light-reflecting color of eye shadow on the center of the eyelid, then blend slightly. When you are blinking, the peek-a-boo effect of the spotlight will draw attention to your eyes.

16. To prevent lip color from sticking to the teeth, put your index finger in your mouth, close your lips around it and pull your finger out. Any excess lip color will stick to the skin on your finger and not on your teeth.

17. Lip color can do, in a pinch, for blush or eye shadow if blended correctly. Just rub a little on your finger and apply to the eyes and cheeks, and blend, baby, blend.

18. If your eye shadow looks a little too dark, try adding some facial powder over the top with your eye shadow brush.

19. If you are applying a lash thickener, be sure to allow the product to completely dry before applying mascara, to avoid clumps.

20. Every glamour girl needs at least one red lipstick stashed in her beauty bag. Red is the one color that is timeless and classic yet sexy and chic at the same time.

21. Blush is the one makeup product that you will never have to change. Find one that you adore, looks adorable on you, and you're set for life.

22. To set your makeup, lightly spritz the face with mineral water, or spray mineral water onto a sea sponge and lightly press the sponge into the skin, without rubbing. Allow to dry. Makeup will last and last.

23. Apply your blush lightly before applying your eye makeup and lip color. More can be added later if needed; however, putting too much blush before eye and lip colors could make you overcompensate, making the eye makeup and lip color darker. Keep it in balance.

24. Facial tissues are what makeup dreams are made of. They can be called upon to blot lip color, to clean up over-loaded mascara wands, or, when pressed into the skin after the application of foundation, to absorb any excess oil from the product that will affect its staying power.

25. Color correctors can be applied under foundation to alter your skin tone. If you are very ruddy, opt for green color corrector. If you are sallow, lilac can brighten up your complexion. Use color correctors sparingly and blend so that they go undetected.

26. For nighttime drama, decide to make either the eyes or the lips the focal point of your face. If you try to accentuate both, the results can look dated, harsh, and fake. If it is the eyes you are going to play up, then use just a wash of color on the lips. If a dramatic lip color is your desire, then neutral eye shadow is the way to go.

27. Make eyeliner application easier by slightly lifting your eyelid at the eyebrow with one finger, so that the skin is taut. The eyeliner will glide on. Be sure not to pull the skin to the excess. Just a tiny tug will do it.

28. Sample before you buy. Most cosmetic companies offer samples of their products. Ask for some, or check their Web sites for any sample offers. Try them for a few days to see how they look and feel on your skin. If you like them, buy them. If you don't, well, you just saved yourself the trouble of returning them.

29. Before going to a big event, give yourself a dress rehearsal. Practice by applying your look beforehand, and see how it looks and feels. True glamour girls test-drive before hitting the road.

30. Eyeglasses can distort your eyes and your eye makeup. Nearsighted lenses have a tendency to make the eyes appear smaller. To counteract this reduction, opt for brighter, bolder shadows and lots of mascara to ensure that your eyes will not disappear. If you are farsighted, lenses can make your eyes look bigger and your eye makeup more prominent. Opt for more muted colors that will be less obvious. Check out the newer glass styles. Ask your optician which style makes your eyes shine bright.

PART 4

THE
THRIFTY
GIRL'S
GUIDE TO A
GLAMOROUS
BODY

This section will cover body basics. From cellulite to hair removal, nail care to fragrance, I'll help you make the most of your beautiful body. There are a million low-cost methods to keep you looking great, from head to toe!

Chapter Sixteen

Body Beautiful

" Each body has its art.... "

—GWENDOLYN BROOKS

How the body moves, stands, sits, caresses, dresses, and is cared for tells the world whether it is loved, hated, or just plain tolerated. There probably isn't a woman alive who cannot find fault with her body. Even super-models and celebrities are quoted daily as to which body part or parts they consider their personal flaws.

Finding fault with the body does not help anything. In fact, finding fault and concentrating on the less than perfect parts of the body does nothing to improve mood, esteem, or confidence. Instead, all fault finding does is create feelings of insecurity and self-loathing, and instills a body picture in the mind of despair, or "what's the use." Who really wants to go around the rest of their lives loathing anything—especially their own body parts? Instead, decide that a new mind-set of acceptance and what is beautiful needs to occur. Consider it like a Glamour Girl twelve-step program for the body. Decide here and now to change the things about your body that you can change, learn to accept the things about your body that you cannot change, and have the wisdom to know the difference.

THE SCOOP ON STATISTICS

A recent ad for the Body Shop proclaimed, "There are over three billion women who don't look like supermodels and only eight who do." Ain't that the truth? Here's the real skinny on the stats:

AVERAGE WOMAN: Height 5'4"; size 12; bust 37"; waist 29"; and hips 40".

AVERAGE MANNEQUIN: Height 6'; size 6; bust 34"; waist 23": and hips 34".

NAOMI CAMPBELL: Height 5'10"; size 6; bust 34"; waist 23"; and hips 34".

BARBIE (IF A REAL WOMAN): Height 7'2"; size less than zero; bust 44"; waist 22"; and hips 36".

Not only are Barbie's vital statistics physiologically impossible, her neck is twice the length of that of a normal human being. The vital statistics for mannequins are so extreme that a living woman who could boast the equivalent measurements would have too little body fat to menstruate. And for what's its worth, today's typical model weighs 20 percent less than the average woman. Ten years ago, the difference for the model was only 10 percent less.

INTRODUCE YOURSELF

From the neck up, we know our skin like the back of our hands, but our bodies often go unnoticed—or worse—forgotten. This chapter is about taking the time to introduce yourself to you. Check out the skin on your body with as much care as you do your face. A sure way to love yourself is to enjoy your uniqueness. Polish and smooth the skin, bathe in luxury, slather on body moisturizing creams, and surround yourself with a delicious fragrance that says, "I am special, and I enjoy being me."

CLEANSING

Although the skin on the body is thicker and hardier than facial skin, it too, needs tender loving care. So many skin problems, such as dry, flaky, or itchy skin, are due to what is used to cleanse the body skin. In every tub and shower soap dish is a bar of soap. While soap is a fast and easy way to clean the skin, the kind of soap determines the look and feel of your skin.

The Ideal Bar of Soap

A good soap should leave your skin feeling and smelling fresh. It should not leave any greasy residue, nor should it clog your pores. Leaving the skin feeling fresh is different from being squeaky clean. Skin that "squeaks" is a sure sign that the skin has been totally stripped of oil—overcleansed, and the main cause of dry surface skin.

The best soap choice is a French milled vegetable-based soap. Vegetable soaps contain ingredients that will gently cleanse the skin, while at the same time caressing the skin with essential oils. Lavender, rosemary, sweet almond, and citrus all are wonderful for the body and, with their heavenly aromas, good for the soul as well. You don't have to break the bank to buy these soaps, either. You can find these soaps in the soap aisle of your regular drugstore.

Body Wash

Body washes are wonderful ways to add a little spa experience into your daily wash-and-go whirlwind days. Body washes come in all types of formulas and fragrances—some are even scented in your signature fragrance. Try these low-cost brands:

- Hydromiel Honey Shower Cream
- St. Ive's Energizing Citrus

Washes are easy to use. Squeeze about the size of a nickel in the hand or on a washcloth and cover the body. Rinse, and you are done. With such a small amount of body wash needed, you won't be washing your money down the drain.

Step Away from the Deodorant Soap

Deodorant soaps are the most drying of all soaps and are not usually necessary for a culture that bathes the way we do. Unless you are running a marathon or working up a huge sweat another way, a regular cleansing soap or wash will do just as good a job and be less irritating to the skin. Also, deodorant soaps are designed to eliminate odors—all odors, even good ones. If you find that your fragrance doesn't linger like it used to, check to see if your cleansing product contains deodorant ingredients.

Bathing Versus Showering

Showering is the quickest and most popular way, hands down, to clean the skin. With the morning mad dash, showers for the most part are simply a means to an end. Wash and go, so you can go. But they can also be five-minute havens for treating yourself to an inexpensive beauty bonus now and then. While your hair is conditioning, apply your exfoliating product. While shaving your legs, apply a deep conditioner to your hair. Apply a facial mask before entering the shower and allow the shower steam to work wonders on the mask while you shower as usual. Plus, rinsing a mask off in the shower is so easy. Just put your face under the warm (not hot) water stream while you use circular motions on the skin to remove.

THROW IN THE TOWEL

For an all-over, spring-your-body-back-to-life feeling, grab a towel. Instead of the same pat dry after bathing, briskly rub your entire body with a terry cloth towel. The brisk rub back and forth stimulates the blood flow and revives even the most sluggish skins. You will feel alive, your circulation will increase, and your skin will glow all over.

The art of the bath is such a wonderful experience, you need to experience it more! The bath provides time to relax, rejuvenate, and revive yourself. Bathing is one way to turn off the world and truly focus on you. One way to start feeling good in your skin is to take a long, languorous soak in a tub surrounded by candles, music, and a closed door.

You can put salts, bubbles, or oils into your bath. The decision is yours, and all these are available for a reasonable price. There is something about a bubble bath with a glass of champagne that brings out the Glamour Girl in us all.

For a tried and true spa bath, do as the French do and try a Thalassotherapy treatment. Thalassotherapy, which features treatments using seawater, has been around for centuries but is now the current trend in spa treatments. For almost nothing, you can create a detoxifying, bloat-banishing bath spa treatment that would cost a tidy sum at the spa. Add one cup of Epsom salts to a warm bath. Soak for at least fifteen minutes. If the water begins to cool, add more hot water. Epsom salts, like seawater, contain magnesium chloride, which aids in drawing out excess fluids. Be sure to drink plenty of water after this treatment, as water will help to continue flushing your system and will keep the bloating away.

EXFOLIATING

Soaps and washes clean away the daily dirt and grime. Exfoliating products are designed to remove excess dead skin and stimulate blood flow to the skin. Exfoliators help the circulatory and lymphatic systems release waste and speed up cell renewal.

Skin that has been exfoliated absorbs moisturizers better, relieves skin itchiness, and, over time, produces skin that has a healthy glow. For the best results, exfoliate the entire body (not the face) with a quality exfoliator once a week during the colder months, and twice a week during the summer.

Exfoliating Tools

Washcloths, loofahs, sea sponges, scrubbies, and exfoliating mitts will help the exfoliating product work more effectively. Some cosmetic companies have exfoliating soaps. The soap either will contain ingredients that help remove dead skin cells, or are made with the soap on one side of the bar while the other side is made from a loofah-type material.

Exfoliating products contain ingredients such as salts, crushed nut meats or oatmeal, seaweed, and other grainy materials. Found in jars, bottles, and in dry form, all are very simple to use. First wet the skin, apply the product either directly or with an exfoliating aid like a washcloth, and gently glide the product over the body, allowing the product to do the work. Do not apply extra pressure, as to do so could result in skin irritation. Be sure to apply to the bottom of the feet—taking care to remove the product carefully so as not to slip. Rinse and pat the skin dry.

Just about every cosmetic company makes a scrub product. It is just a matter of choice as to fragrant or fragrant free, liquid, cream, or dry. An easy and thrifty way to make a spa-quality treatment scrub at home is to mix two tablespoons of Dead Sea salt (found at the grocery store next to the table salt) and one cup of olive oil. Shower as usual, and then while still in the shower, gently rub the body with the mixture. Rinse, and rinse again. The Dead Sea salt contains minerals that will help loosen dead skin, while the olive oil, with its monounsaturated fat, will moisturize and soften.

Dry brushing the skin is another way to exfoliate the skin. Used since the time of Cleopatra, it is a super modern way to keep dry, flaky skin away for good. Use a natural-fiber bath brush that has a handle attachment to reach your back. Before bathing, while the skin is dry, begin dry brushing at the toes, feet, ankles, and legs. Work up the body, always in the direction of the heart. Continue up the torso, stomach, back, and arms. All it takes is about five to seven gentle, long brush strokes over each area. Allow the motion to do the work—gentle brushing is best. The movement is similar to that of shaving. Start dry brushing two or three times a week until your skin begins to feel very soft to the touch. To maintain softness, dry brush once a week. Shower as usual after brushing, pat dry, and add a bit of moisture. You will find that you actually use less moisturizer as time goes on. This is because the skin will be more efficient at producing it from the inside.

MOISTURIZING

The skin on the body takes a lot of wear and tear. It is always—well, almost always, covered with clothing. Clothing that rubs back and forth puts ingredients such as detergent, fabric softeners, and dry cleaning fluid on nearly every skin cell. Moisturizing the skin protects it from invaders like these and more. While the skin is very forgiving, treating it with a little respect and a big drink of moisture every day will do wonders for your overall body satisfaction—to say nothing about how good it feels. Skin that is silky smooth and radiant just has a glow.

SLOW DOWN

Since bathing time for the most part is at warp speed, most of us want hand and body creams that sink in fast. But the truth is, the faster the formula absorbs, the more it could actually be drying the skin at the same time. What makes a cream penetrate quickly is alcohol. Choose a slower absorbing formula—one without alcohol, for the richest and most nourishing benefits. So it takes a minute or so longer to rub it in; think of the long-term benefits to smoother, more supple skin. You will see that it's worth the wait.

The type of moisturizer you should use depends on your skin condition. Drier skins love a moisturizer that is thick and rich with emollients. Oilier skins like a light coating of a liquid moisturizer. Normal skins can choose what they like. The main thing is: apply it regularly! For the best results, remember the three-minute rule. After you bath and dry, you have about three minutes before the skin begins to close the pores. Applying moisturizer within three minutes after bathing allows for better absorption where the thirsty cells need it most.

It is not necessary to break the bank for a good-quality moisturizer. Drugstores carry excellent brands that will do the job beautifully. Find one that you like and use it after every bath.

For added fun, some formulas now contain ingredients that add a little color to the skin via a sunless tanning method. The color is deposited gradually, so it looks natural, not fake. Now you can look like you have been on holiday, without leaving town. That's what I call an imitation vacation.

HAIR REMOVAL

Since ancient times, women have been fighting Mother Nature in pursuit of smooth, baby-soft, hair-free skin. There are plenty of methods out there, but the best method for keeping extra hair away has yet to be discovered. Of all of the ways to remove hair, here are the most popular.

Shaving

Shaving's benefits are that it is easy, fast, and cheap. The downside is that you will have to shave every day if you want totally smooth skin, or every other day if you can live with the tiny stubble. It is best for legs and underarms. There is no pain in shaving, unless, of course, you nick yourself. Keeping a fresh shaver will help lessen the drag of the razor, and therefore decrease nicks. Tips:

- Wait two to three minutes after getting into the shower or bath before shaving, to soften hairs.
- Apply steady, light pressure and change the blades every five or six shaves.

- Use water or oil rather than soap, which leaves the skin overly dry and taut.

Depilatories

Depilatories are creams, gels, or lotions designed for hair removal. These are inexpensive and long-lasting, lasting between five and fifteen days, depending on regrowth rate (two weeks is average). The cons are that they can be messy, sometimes smelly, and time-consuming, as formulas can take up to ten minutes or more to work. Depilatories are best used on legs, underarms, bikini area, and facial hair (its formula is designed for facial use). There is no pain with this method, unless you leave the product on too long or you have a sensitivity to the ingredients. It is best to do a spot test when trying a depilatory.

When using depilatories, rinse off with cool water as opposed to warm (never hot), and avoid sunscreen, body lotions, and self-tanners for at least two hours to prevent irritation.

Waxing

Waxing produces silky smooth skin that lasts for weeks. Little fine hairs begin to emerge after a couple of weeks, and thicker growth in about three to four weeks. Hair actually becomes finer, and in some cases, less hair returns with repeated use. Waxing can be done at home, if you are skilled and patient. Day spas are another option but can be costly. The best method is to have it professionally done, watch the treatment techniques closely, and then purchase an at-home kit. Waxing is best for legs, bikini area, underarms, upper lip, and eyebrows. The cons of waxing are that it is messy, time-consuming, and painful—at least for a few seconds! Tips:

- Hold the skin taut before the wax is pulled. Remove the wax in the opposite direction from the growth of the hair.

- Gently pat the area just waxed to soften the zing of the sting.
- Allow a few days between waxing and sun exposure, as newly exposed areas are more sensitive.
- If hair is long, trim it with scissors so the wax will not matte or break the hair off halfway.
- Read the directions and follow them to the letter. Some formulas are safe to use to rewax an area if you need to; others are not designed to reapply.

Bleaching

If your "wild hairs" are not so wild, bleaching is one way to camouflage their existence. This is best used for facial hair, dark hair on forearms, or shins, if you are lucky enough not to have much extra hair there. The downside of bleaching is that it is time-consuming, messy, and impractical for larger areas. There is no pain with bleaching, unless the product is left on too long. Always do a patch test to see how your skin and hair reacts and looks after bleaching.

Sugaring

This method dates back more than 2,000 years to the Middle East. The technique is similar to waxing, but because the paste sticks to the hair rather than the skin, it is a little less painful than waxing. Sugaring can be used on all areas of the body. The cons are that it is messy, and there is a risk of ingrown hairs with this method.

Find a professional to do the treatment for the first time so that when you do the treatment at home you will be familiar with how it is applied and removed and what care needs to happen afterward.

CELLULITE

The bottom line is that more than 85 percent of women have some form of cellulite somewhere on their bodies. While it is somewhat comforting to know if you are in the percentage majority, in this case misery does not love company. Women are prone to cellulite because of the way our connective fibers are arranged in our bodies. While men's connective tissue runs at an angle, women's tissues run more vertically. Also, our hormones, which make our hips, thighs, and bums curvier, also add to the cellulite plan.

Cellulite forms when the fat cells within the connective tissue enlarge, which restricts blood and lymph flow circulation. Excess toxins then build up, as well as fluids, which swell the fat cells. Not pretty, indeed. You can diminish the look of cellulite by coupling a healthy eating plan with exercise. You know the drill: avoid fatty and junk foods, drink plenty of water, limit alcohol beverages, and get plenty of exercise.

For extra measure, you can topically apply cellulite creams to the areas to reduce the appearance of the cellulite. These creams usually contain natural ingredients such as horse chestnut, ivy, and caffeine to boost your circulation.

THRIFTY TIP

You can make cellulite creams doubly effective by massaging them thoroughly into the skin with your fingertips.

Some cellulite creams come with their own plastic or rubber hand-held mitts to help boost the circulation. The key is dedication. An active anti-cellulite plan needs to include all of the above things as well as a strict schedule for a daily regime of use.

For an effective home cellulite remedy, use aromatherapy. Aromatherapy has been found to be very effective for treating cellulite. There are a number of ready-blended oils on the market designed for the fight against cellulite.

THRIFTY TIP

You can easily make your own aromatherapeutic blended oils to fight cellulite. Simply add 2 drops each of rosemary and fennel essentials oils to 1 tablespoon of a carrier oil (like almond or sesame). Massage this mixture thoroughly into the affected areas every day after you bathe.

The number one body-beautiful beauty tip is free: be confident. Confidence is smart, sexy, and sassy. Learn to shine with your confidence, and not only will everyone totally believe that you are gorgeous and glamorous, but you will appear even younger than your years. Strut your stuff—confidently. Remember to love the skin you are in. After all, it has to last you a lifetime!

Chapter Seventeen

Scent of a Woman

66 A woman is never well-dressed without perfume. 99

—COCO CHANEL

Fragrance is both very private, as the essence of perfume mixes with the essence of your body oils, and very public, as your chosen scent wafts out to the world, creating an olfactory signature of sorts. Your head-to-toe style of dress creates a statement of who you are, and it is your fragrance that punctuates your statement.

TOP DRAWER

If you like the smell of the magazine fragrance rub-on, tear out the page and put it in your delicates drawer. Another good use is to keep a couple of the pages in your closet, one on the top shelf and another where you store your shoes.

More than 110 new scents are launched each year. You only have to open any women's magazine for your nose to be completely overwhelmed with all of the perfume ads and rub-on samples (there's a way to get free perfume!). Visit your local department store on a Saturday and just try to make it down the fragrance aisle without getting spritzed by one of the cosmetic companies' fragrance models. No wonder it has been said that picking out a new fragrance is "nose-boggling."

While perfumes are not a department in which to be overly thrifty—there is nothing worse than smelling cheap—this chapter will cover how to maximize your scent once you have sprayed it, and how to keep your perfumes fresher, longer.

UNDER THE NOSE

Never rush into a decision regarding a new scent—doing so will only result in wasted perfume and money. Several factors need to go into the olfactory decision. The perfect perfume takes time to find. Do not be too impulsive when purchasing a new fragrance. Just because your favorite celebrity wears it, or the fact that the packaging is exactly the same color as your dressing area are not good reasons to choose it. While fragrance is an emotional experience, the purchase needs to be a physical one.

Fragrance is constructed in the form of an imaginary pyramid, with top, middle and base notes.

Top Notes

Top notes hit you when you open the bottle and spray it onto your skin. They are short bursts of fresh, green, and zesty notes that you notice immediately. They last for a very short time, fading in about ten minutes. Citrus, peach, bergamot, and black currant are common top notes.

Middle Notes

Middle notes, also known as the heart and soul notes, describe the smells that evolve after the first ten minutes of exposure on the skin. Middle notes have a flowery bouquet and are an important part of the fragrance because they last between two and four hours. This scent is why you purchase the fragrance. Popular middle note scents are rose, jasmine, gardenia, lilac, ylang ylang, tuberose, and lily of the valley.

Base Notes

Base notes are the smells that slowly develop to hold the whole fragrance together and that will linger longest. Some base notes are amber, musk, sandalwood, patchouli, and vetiver.

THRIFTY TIP

Only purchase a fragrance when you like the base notes; you (and everyone else around you) will smell for these the remainder of the wearing.

Time changes everything. The spritz that you put on your skin at the store will not be the scent that you smell later on during the day. With the top, middle, and base notes mixing with your personal chemical composition, the fragrance will evolve, so take your time in deciding, unless you want another bottle gathering dust on your dressing table.

HOW TO PICK THE PERFECT PERFUME

With fragrance terms such as *floral*, *ozonic*, *fougere*, and *chypre* to describe the scent, no wonder we are confused. What do those terms have to do with how it smells? All fragrance—no matter what the brand, Coco to Chantilly, Pleasures to Poison— all belong to one of five fragrance families.

Floral

Florals are the oldest fragrance family. In ancient times, fragrances consisted of rose and lavender scents. Modern florals contain many different flowers as a base. Flowers such as lily, carnation, hyacinth, sweet pea, and other springtime bouquets make up today's floral family. Florals are the safest scent to wear, as they rarely overpower and are usually delicate in strength.

Fougere

Fougere means "fern" in French. *Fougere* is an invented term, as ferns do not smell. The category became popular in the late 1800s when a perfumer mixed a floral scent with something made in the laboratory that was an imitation of a scent occurring in nature. The natural scent and the manufactured scent were combined, and the end result was very different and interesting to smell. Fougeres are one of the biggest sellers in the world of fragrance, as today's technology of combining real with imaginary smells is seemingly limitless.

Chypre

Chypres scents are found in nature. Smells come from the forest and in the mossy woods. A classic chypre scent contains oak moss, musk, or sandalwood and is then mixed with floral essences of rose or jasmine, among others. The end result is a fresh, clean, yet sensual and earthy combination.

Oriental

Orientals are the sexiest of perfumes and also the headiest. The scents smell of exotic places and spices. Orientals are also the longest lasting fragrances, so less can, and in most cases should, be used when applying from the oriental fragrance family. Hints of ambergris along with woody, spicy tones are often mixed with nuances of fresh flowers to add depth and mystery to the fragrance.

Ozonic

Ozonics scents are the newest types of fragrances. Known as aroma chemicals, they evoke the smell of a picnic, a watermelon, or outdoor smells such as salt water and an ocean breeze. In the natural response category, you either love these fragrances or you can *definitely* leave them.

FRAGRANCE COLLAGE

Perfume experts have created a series of fragrance collages that allow you to use what you like tactilely and visually to direct you toward a fragrance category that most closely matches your style.

Classic

The look of orchids, Greek-style architecture, crisp white color, and rich leather typically appeal to those who enjoy classic scents. Scents that are rich yet subtle and elegant will work well with classic tastes. Examples of classic scents include:

- Chanel No. 5
- Lancôme Poeme
- Worth Je Reviens
- Lanvin Arpege

Glamorous

Those who gravitate toward glamorous scents will be intrigued by birds of paradise, exotic flowers, buildings with curves in the design, true reds, and the look and feel of fur against the skin. Scents with sensuality, with a flair for the dramatic, are considered glamorous. Examples of glamorous scents include:

- Chanel Coco
- Jean Patou 1000
- Salvador Dali Eau de Dali
- YSL Opium

Modern

Fuchsia-colored roses, architecture that combines curves with straight angles, and the feel of velvet are connected with modern scents. Upbeat fragrances are designed for this category. Examples of modern scents include:

- Estee Lauder Beautiful
- Tiffany Trueste
- Giorgio Giorgio

Natural

Natural scents evoke images of day lilies, farmhouses, the color blue, and suede. Naturals love the outdoors and innocent fresh air scents. Examples include:

- Estee Lauder Pleasures
- YSL Paris
- Chanel Allure
- Cacharel Anais Anais

Casual

Those who gravitate toward casual scents are typically intrigued by wildflowers, seaside towns, the color pink, and the look and feel of linen against the skin. Casuals are stylish yet considered easy-to-wear fragrances. Examples include:

- Chanel No. 22
- 4711
- YSL Rive Gauche

Romantic

Romantics typically enjoy daisies in every color, lace of any kind, and clean crisp white clapboard houses. Romantic scents are a mix of flowers, spices, and fruits. Examples are:

- Gucci Accenti
- Caron Nocturnes
- Christian Dior Dolce Vita

HOW DO I SMELL?

Within a few minutes of your trying a fragrance on, the nose becomes acclimated to the scent and begins losing the scent gradually. Unless you are deliberately holding an area you spritzed with perfume up to your nose, you will lose the ability to smell it shortly. This is not the case with those around you. Whatever you can smell, those around you can smell more. Trying on several fragrances to test and then going back to the office may get you more attention than you want. Save the power testing for days when you can take advantage of the great outdoors.

You can spritz a little extra on a perfume blotter or cotton ball from the perfume counter to keep in your purse to test the fragrance throughout the day and dab onto the skin now and then.

THRIFTY TIP

If you want a scented body cream or lotion, simply add a drop or a spritz of your fragrance in with your application of body cream or lotion. You can also take a small container of cream or lotion and add a few drops, gently swirl to mix and ta-da—perfumed perfection!

The strength of scent you wear controls the distance it can be smelled from and how long it will last. If the fragrance is alcohol-based such as cologne, eau de parfum, and eau de toilette, it will fade quickly at first and then level off. Oil- and cream-based perfumes such as perfume, body creams, and bath oils, when worn as perfume, will taper off more gradually throughout the day.

- Colognes typically last one to four hours.
- Eau de toilette and eau de parfum usually last from four to six hours.
- Body lotion or body cream lasts from three to eight hours.
- Perfume lasts the longest, from five to eight hours.

Layering the fragrance allows the fragrance to last longer, as it wears over time, rather than putting too much on at the onset with overspraying. By using companion products like bath washes/oils, body lotions/creams, or bath powder, and *then* spraying your fragrance, you will smell wonderful all day, without overpowering yourself or others.

PROTECTING YOUR INVESTMENT

Knowing how to store and care for your fragrance will allow you to enjoy its true essence for a longer run. Air, heat, and light are a fragrance nightmare. Here are some "common scents" tips to maximize your fragrance wardrobe:

- An unopened bottle of fragrance will usually keep safely for three years, provided it has been kept properly away from heat and light.
- Open fragrances have about a year-and-a-half to two-year shelf life. When the scent begins to smell slightly of vinegar, becomes darker, or sticky/greasy when applied, it is time to part ways.
- Limiting yourself to two open fragrances at a time will allow you to use the product up quickly, before it changes scents.
- Bathrooms are not good areas to keep fragrances, as the constant warm steam will cause the product to break down faster.
- Keeping the fragrances in the refrigerator will allow them to last longer. Plus, they feel great on a warm summer day.
- If you have a larger bottle of fragrance, pour some into a small atomizer to use, and keep the rest in the refrigerator for safekeeping.

Quick Notes on Fragrance

- If you have sprayed too much perfume and taking a quick bath is not an option, dilute the scent by rubbing with a warm, soapy washcloth on the areas you put it.
- High altitudes decrease the longevity of perfume as well as the potency of its aroma. You might need to add a little more to last.
- Fragrance doesn't last as long on dry skin as it does on oilier skins.
- Some perfumes smell stronger on someone who eats a lot of spicy or high-fat foods.
- Be careful where you spray the body if planning time in the sun. Alcohol from the fragrance can cause a sunburn where skin is exposed.
- Wait a few minutes after bathing to apply your perfume. Warm water causes the pores to dilate, temporarily leaving skin more sensitive to any product applied directly after bathing.
- Women have a better sense of smell than men, especially during the first half of the menstrual cycle.
- Everyone has a "fragrance fingerprint." How you smell with any fragrance is dependent on heredity, complexion, and diet.

It's totally up to you to decide whether you want to change fragrances like you change your clothes or to have a signature fragrance. The main thing to remember is to be memorable. Leave them wanting more!

Chapter Eighteen

Helping Hands

"To keep your hands smooth and lovely, put two things in the dish-water—someone else's hands."

—UNKNOWN

Hands and nails are very visible indicators of age and lifestyle. Smooth skin and manicured nails tell the world that you take yourself seriously. Whether you talk with your hands or not—they are speaking loud and clear all the same.

Hands are always on display. Your facial complexion may say one thing while your hands say another. To help your hands say beautiful things about you is not as hard as it would seem. Hands are great responders to a little loving care and will thank you with smoother, firmer, and more translucent skin in a snap!

You need to know that the skin on the hands is thinner. It has less wrinkle- and vein-hiding ability as the hands have less fat and moisturizing oil glands. On average, the hands have only 100 glands per square inch compared to the facial skin, which averages over 900 per inch. With their limited amount of oil glands it is no wonder that our hands are the first parts that prune in the bath water.

In addition to having limited oil glands, our hands are virtually exposed to the elements and left unprotected nearly all of the time. Think about the sun exposure that the back of the hands get just by holding onto a steering wheel, when plunged into hot soapy water "just to wash a glass or two," or when quickly dashing here or there in winter without donning gloves, and, of course, think how hands are used as tools when trying to pry something open or scrape something off. Can you imagine treating your face that way?

Thrifty Girls, it is time to raise your hand and take a vow to love, honor, and protect your hands and nails from this day forward. Here are a few simple, easy-to-do tips that will have your hands applauding in no time.

HANDS-LOVING REGIME

Just like skin, hair, and body care regimes keep you on the beauty and glamour track, steps are needed to make your hands look and feel their most beautiful best.

> **CLEANSE.** Choose hand soap carefully. Extra-strength and antibacterial soaps strip the oils from the hands and cause them to look dry, flaky, and irritated. Instead opt for a gentle liquid hand soap that has skin conditioners and essential oils in the ingredients.

> **EXFOLIATE.** Just as you remove the dry, dead skin cells from the face, neck, décolleté and body, treat your hands to an exfoliation treatment as well. Add a little of your facial exfoliating product to the back of the hands while you are doing your facial treatment. Rinse and pat dry.

MASK. Facial masks make an excellent instant pick-me-up for the hands. As you are applying your facial mask, put the remainder on the back of hands. Leave on for ten minutes. Rinse and pat dry.

MOISTURIZE. At least twice a day (and always after washing your hands), apply moisturizer to the hands. Hands that are dry, cracked, or chapped are not only uncomfortable but also more prone to infection, as bacteria can get into the tiny cracks. Keep them hydrated.

SUNSCREEN. Exposure to the sun accelerates aging on the hands tremendously. Showing up as age or liver spots, these spots are tell-tale signs that sun damage has occurred. Regular use of a good sunscreen—minimum SPF of 15—will prevent brown spots by at least 85 percent.

PROTECT. Protecting the hands from harsh elements such as dishwater or housecleaning agents with rubber gloves is a must. When you are working in the yard, garden gloves should be worn as well.

NAIL IT

Nail bars and manicure spas can now be found on almost every corner of the block. The concept came from New York City, where manicures are an important part of many women's weekly routine. These women know that attractive hands and nails make you feel pretty, and well-groomed nails accessorize any outfit, to say nothing of the wonderful "I'm worth it" feeling that treating yourself to a manicure gives.

Here is everything you need to know to give yourself an oh-so-glamorous makeover in the comfort of your own home.

Manicure Makeover

- Begin by removing nail polish and/or oils from the nail bed by applying a polish remover. An easy way to remove nail polish is to soak a cotton ball with polish remover. Place the ball on the nail and hold in place for about ten seconds. The nail polish will become soft, allowing for an easier removal.

- File nails to desired shape with an emery board. File in one direction only, parallel to the nail bed. Do not curve into the corner of the nail. (Metal nail files are too harsh and cause the nail to weaken or crack.)

- Allow nails on each hand to soak in a bowl of gentle anti-bacterial soapy water for five minutes. Add a couple of drops of your favorite essential oil to hydrate the skin and to enjoy the aroma. Remove and pat dry the hands.

- Clean gently under nails with a file. Lightly is the key word. Don't gouge the skin underneath.

- Apply cuticle oil and push cuticles back with an orange stick, or cuticle pusher. Massage the cuticle oil into the skin and nail bed.

- Buff the nail beds with a nail buffer to create a smooth area on which to polish. Buff just enough to make the nail bed look rosy. Don't overbuff, as you will stress the nail.

- Put a bit of polish remover on a cotton ball and gently swipe each nail bed to remove any leftover cuticle oil from the nail before polishing.
- Apply nail base coat. Let dry for three minutes.
- Apply two coats of your favorite polish, allowing three to four minutes between coats to dry.
- Apply top coat to add shine, protect the nails, and allow the color to last longer.
- Allow twenty minutes for nails to dry and be completely set.

Plan on penciling in your calendar your manicure makeover session on a weekly basis. Manicures are easy add-ons to other beauty routines that you have already planned—like while your hair color is processing, your feet are soaking in a pedicure, or your facial mask is working—use the extra minutes to do your nails. Combining beauty treatments is easy when you plan ahead.

Nail Facts
- Fingernails grow about 1 mm (0.0394 in) each week.
- It takes three to four months for a fingernail to renew itself from base to tip, and six to seven months for the entire fingernail to regrow.
- Growth can be slowed dramatically by illness, poor eating habits, or dieting.
- Stress can increase growth to such rapid speeds that the nail cannot keep up and will break, crack, and peel at a moment's notice.
- Nails grow faster on the dominant hand. This is because the additional activity stimulates the circulation.
- Nails also grow faster in the warm weather months and just before your period.
- Aging slows down the growth of the nail.

Nail Tips

- When going to a manicurist, do not put yourself at risk of infection from someone else's germs, bacteria, or fungus—bring your own manicure kit with you, or leave a personal kit with your manicurist to be stored exclusively for you.

- To fast-dry your nails, dip your nails into ice water. Ice water speeds up the hardening process.

- Always use acetone-free polish remover, which will not strip vital oils from nails. Look for "gentle" or "non-drying" on the label.

- If you want a "scents-ery" experience, instead of soaking your hands in just soapy water, add a spritz of your favorite perfume to the water. Your hands will be soaking, while your fragrance is adding to your personal glamour.

- If polish removal around the cuticle is difficult, use an orange stick with the tip wrapped in a piece of cotton, dipped in nail polish remover, to gently remove excess polish from the stubborn areas.

- Fast-dry topcoats, and quick-dry sprays while drying the nails quickly, will add to the nail's chip factor. Decide to allow your nails to dry naturally for the longest lasting manicure.

- Keeping the polish light and neutral will allow the longest wear, as chips and nicks do not show as much.

- Celebrities and socialites agree: keep it mild on the hands and wild on the toes, keeping classic neutral shades on the hands makes it easy to coordinate clothing. Plus, mild colors allow the attention to be on you—not your nails. Keep the wild colors for the toes to peek out of sandals.

- To keep fingernails and the delicate cuticle skin healthy and hydrated, put cuticle oil, vitamin E, or almond oil on them every day. Keep a bottle on your desk at work or beside your favorite chair so that you will be reminded to rub a little on. Also apply a coating of the oil before swimming to protect the cuticles from the pool chlorine. It just takes two minutes, but what a difference it makes.

Well-groomed hands should be part of every woman's beauty routine. Spending one-half hour on your hands a week will pay off in a week's worth of feeling confident, beautiful, and glamorous. Now that's what I call a good return on your investment!

Chapter Nineteen
Sole Survivor

" When a woman is dressed to kill, her feet are usually the first victims. "

—UNKNOWN

Happy feet make for a happy woman. When your feet are killing you, it shows on every part of your body and most especially your face. No matter how fabulous the shoes, pinched and cramped toes are just not worth it, plain and simple. Plus, think about slipping out of your oh-so-fabulous shoes and revealing a "discount" looking foot. Kind of ruins the image, don't you think?

Take a look at your feet right now. Are you happy with what you see? Are they smooth, hydrated, and beautifully manicured? Or do they show signs of wear and tear? Are they calloused? Do they have corns, hard patches of skin, or raggedy nails?

RUBBER BAND SNAP

To strengthen and stretch out the toes, place a thick, moderately stiff rubber band around your big toes and pull your feet away from each other slowly. Hold the stretch for five to ten seconds. Repeat ten to twenty times. This is a marvelous way to ease toe cramping and the ouch of bunions.

Feet and toenails truly take a beating. Feet absorb the stress of up to twice your body weight with each and every step. During the average lifetime, over 70,000 miles are walked—that is four times around the earth! Coupled with the fact that on average over 9,000 steps are taken every day, it is a wonder our feet have not given us our marching orders!

BLISTERS AWAY

Petroleum jelly lightly rubbed over the entire foot will eliminate friction and prevent blisters. Also, hosiery is not as likely to get a run because of skin snagging.

The good news is that feet, like our hands, are quick to forgive and say thanks for the attention they receive. A simple routine of foot pampering now and then is all that is needed to add a little twinkle to your toes and put a little pep in your step.

FOOT FIXES

On average, our feet are stuffed in shoes fifteen hours a day. And depending on the weatheror the occasion, add socks or hosiery to that equation—it is no wonder that the feet can suffer from unpleasant ailments. To help put your feet on the right track, here are a few thrifty tips to remedy the situation.

BLISTERS: Blisters are caused by the accumulation of fluid between the skin's inner and outer layers, brought on by constant friction with socks or shoes. While a blister is not a serious condition, it can become infected if not properly treated. Remedy: Try not to burst the blister if possible. If it does break on its own, put an antiseptic solution on the area and cover with a Band-Aid.

CALLUSES: A callus is skin that is thicker than the surrounding skin. The increase in thickness is caused from continual pressure on the area. The feet are most prone to calluses, as the skin on the feet is four times thicker than that on the body. Calluses, if not treated, will become painful and require professional treatment. Remedy: Begin to gently exfoliate the skin daily in the shower with either a pumice stone or a callus grinder. Be sure to slather on moisturizing cream every morning and evening.

CORNS: Corns are small areas of thick, tough skin that arise as a result of friction with shoes or from the buildup of moisture. Remedy: While it is tempting to try and remove corns yourself with one of the corn removers on the market, it is best not to attempt to cure them yourself as you can inadvertently bring on infection. Make an appointment with a podiatrist to treat it.

BUNIONS: Bunions are usually hereditary but can also be caused by ill-wearing shoes. When the big toe begins to curve toward the side rather than pointing straight up, a bunion situation is most likely the cause. Remedy: To prevent a bunion from becoming worse, wear shoes with a straight inside edge to reduce pressure on the joint—avoid pointy-toe shoes altogether. A podiatrist visit is necessary to determine the next step. Depending on the condition, protective pads, specially designed shoes, or, in extreme cases, surgery could be the treatment.

FUNGAL INFECTIONS: Fungus infections are caused from a number of different bacterias. If the feet feel itchy, the skin is red and irritated, or the toenails become discolored and/or thicken, it could be from a fungal infection. Remedy: Always wash and dry the feet well. A commercially prepared product designed to fight feet fungus can be found at the drug store. However, if the infection is on the toenails, the fungus becomes more difficult to treat. Make an appointment with a podiatrist to determine the best remedy.

After bathing, examine your feet to note any changes and to take care of any little problem before it becomes big. Also trim the toenails regularly, at least once a month. Cut them straight across to prevent the curving corners that can cause ingrown toenails.

Toostie Tips

- Change your shoes often, and if you wear high heels, vary your heel height every day.
- An absorbent foot powder sprinkled in the shoes before wearing will help absorb excess moisture and keep the feet smelling sweet.
- If you suffer from burning feet, spritz the feet with a refreshing mist of water mixed with a few drops of rosemary essential oil to cool and soothe.
- Soothe tired feet in a flash by rubbing Vaporub onto clean, dry feet. Put on cotton socks and put your feet up for a while. Vaporub is a decongestant that cools the skin and soothes aches and pains. It's great for traveling to revive the "tour de feet."
- Keep a golf ball in your desk drawer or beside your favorite chair. Slip off your shoes and rub the foot back and forth over the golf ball for two minutes. It is a tension relieving massage that helps with arch strain, foot cramps, or heel pain. You will feel refreshed in no time!

THE PERFECT PEDICURE

Pedicures are the perfect way to tell your feet thank you for all of the things that they do for you each and every day.

THRIFTY TIP

While getting a professional spa pedicure is like being on cloud nine, if your budget is saying no clouds in sight, a do-it-yourself pedicure can be a slice of heaven as well.

Here is what you will need:

- Nail polish remover
- Cotton balls
- Nail clippers
- Emery board
- Cuticle oil
- Scented bath salts
- Antibacterial soap
- Foot bath or soaking tub
- Foot file or pumice stone
- Nail brush or old toothbrush
- Orange stick or rubber-tipped stick
- Body scrub product
- Towel
- Hydrating hand or foot cream
- Base coat
- Nail color polish
- Top coat

1. Begin by removing old polish and/or body oils from the toenails.

2. Trim toenails and smooth edges with an emery board.

3. Soak feet in a footbath basin filled with warm water and add one cup of scented bath salts and one pump of an antibacterial soap. Soak for ten minutes.

4. Take foot file or pumice stone and gently follow the outline of the feet, concentrating on smoothing rough areas.

5. Wet nail brush or toothbrush with the soapy water; gently clean the toenails and cuticles with the brush.

6. Pat dry. Coat the cuticles with the cuticle oil, then push them back with the orange stick or rubber-tipped stick.

7. Apply a small amount of body scrub to each foot and massage gently. Rinse in tub and pat dry.

8. Massage feet with a moisturizing cream until it is completely absorbed.

9. Soak a cotton ball in nail polish remover and apply to toenails to recleanse them and remove any excess moisturizer from them.

10. Separate the toes with a toe separator or tissue them apart so that the polish will not smear.

11. Apply a base coat. Allow to dry for three minutes.

12. Apply two coats of a wonderful, feel-good polish—the sky is the limit for color. Remember, "wild on the toes!" Allow to dry for three to four minutes between coats.

13. End with a shiny topcoat to protect the nails and allow the pedicure to last all month.

14. Wait at least one hour before putting on shoes or socks. Flip-flops are perfect to wear as your toes dry, and you can admire your handiwork a little longer, to boot!

There is something so fun and feminine about perfectly pedicured feet. Every time your Fantasy Fuchsia or your Drop-Dead Red donned toes slip into some sandals, you will get a kick out of how great they look. And even if it is in the dead of winter, seeing your pampered tootsies peeking out of the bed covers or emerging from a bath full of bubbles will put a smile on your face.

Chapter Twenty

Something to Smile About

" Beauty is power; a smile is its sword. "

—CHARLES READE

There is no doubt that a beautiful smile can open doors for you. A mouth full of healthy, white and bright, well-spaced teeth can be one of your most attractive features. In fact, studies show that a person's teeth and smile are what 65 percent of us notice first about a person. An attractive smile and teeth will almost certainly get you noticed wherever you go, whether it's in the world of business or in social circles.

GIMME TWO

Two minutes of teeth brushing is necessary twice a day to really get the teeth their cleanest. Most people only brush for thirty seconds! Get a kitchen timer and set it for two minutes—if it seems like it takes a lifetime—think about all of the things you were missing in your mouth and leaving on your teeth!

Just as our bodies and faces have different shapes, everyone has a different smile and set of teeth as well. While the size and shape of the mouth is pretty much a permanent fixture on your face, your teeth—color, alignment, and shape—can be altered with the help of a skillful cosmetic dentist, for the extreme changes, or with the help of a couple of cosmetic dental products from the drugstore, for the easy—as well as inexpensive—changes. With all of the technological advances in the dental field, putting up with poor teeth is something that you do not have to contend with—even on a limited budget.

When you look in the mirror, do you like your smile? If you think that your smile can be enhanced, consider this chapter a "smile lift" for your face. Think about it—you would not hesitate to fix a skin breakout. Rather, you would apply the necessary blemish remedy ASAP. Having a bad hair day? As fast as you could, you would attempt to fix it at home. And if you couldn't, you would call your hairstylist and make an appointment to have your style and/or color changed. If your teeth need a little attention, decide now to make the changes—a beautiful smile should last a lifetime.

DAILY CARE

The first and most important step to a radiant smile is right in your bathroom. Your toothbrush, toothpaste, floss, and mouth-wash are the keys to unlocking a glamour grin.

> **BRUSH.** Soft nylon bristles with rounded tips are the best to use. The brush head should be 20 mm (0.8 in) or less. A comfortable grip should also be considered, as you are more likely to brush the necessary two minutes if the brush is easy to hold.
>
> **ELECTRIC BRUSHES.** Electric brushes are excellent, as they can clean the teeth and gums better than hand-held brushes. Electric brushes have been proven to lessen plaque and secondary gum disease, which in itself is a good thing. They leave the teeth cleaner, and fresher than a manual toothbrush will. Budgetwise, compare prices, as they range in cost from under $30 to over $60. It is a good investment when you consider that the toothbrush holder will last for years, while you just replace the brush head.
>
> **TOOTHPASTE.** The sky is the limit on what toothpaste you can choose from—it is literally a matter of taste. There are gels, creams, paste, flavored, unflavored, whitening, anticavity, antibacterial, total this, and supreme that—the important thing to remember is to choose one that you will like to taste and feel each and every day and night.
>
> **FLOSS.** Flossing is something that at least 50 percent of us do not do—yet studies prove that it is the most effective way of fighting plaque and gum disease. Each tooth has five surfaces, and brushing reaches only three of them: the top,

the front, and the back. Flossing goes in between the teeth on both sides, allowing the entire tooth to be cleaned. Floss length of 16 to 18 inches works well. Wrap the floss around each of the middle fingers. Slip the floss between your teeth. Form a U shape against the side of one tooth. Beginning at the gum line, use a gentle rubbing motion to remove the particles of food. Repeat with each adjacent tooth, remembering to wind the floss so that you have a clean section of floss to use with each tooth. What keeps me flossing is a sign in my dentist's office that I noticed years ago that put flossing in perspective: "You don't have to floss all of your teeth—just the ones that you want to keep."

MOUTHWASH. While brushing and flossing are the cornerstones of good oral hygiene, a mouthwash is a useful addition to a healthy mouth regime. Rinsing your mouth thoroughly with mouthwash can help prevent bacteria from accumulating on the gums and teeth base line, which causes gum disease and other oral infections. Choose a mouthwash that has antibacterial properties and a flavor that you are able to face day after day.

The proper way to brush the teeth is by placing the brush against the gum at a 45-degree angle. Strokes should be gentle in toothwide increments. Brush each side and the top. Always remember to brush the tongue to remove any excess bacteria— and to keep the breath smelling sweet.

After brushing, rinse the toothbrush and store it brush side up to dry naturally. Never store your toothbrush in a closed container, as that will encourage bacteria to form. Once a week, clean the toothbrush by pouring a couple of drops of antibacterial mouthwash over it, and allow to dry.

Toothbrushes should be changed every two months. Some brushes have color-coated bristles that fade with each use. When the bristle color has faded halfway, it is time to change.

Keep a couple of extra brushes on hand to be able to change as needed. If you keep a travel kit packed, be sure to change your travel toothbrush regularly. Better to toss than overuse.

Every six months, schedule a visit to your dental hygienist. The hygienist will remove plaque as well as surface stains and give teeth a brightening polish. The hygienist will use an ultrasonic device to remove things that you cannot remove with at-home teeth-cleaning regimen. You will love the look and feel of your teeth and gums.

COSMETIC PROCEDURES

For cases such as straightening teeth, getting fillings, and repairing tooth surfaces, a cosmetic dentist appointment will be necessary. If you live within driving distance to a dental school, you are in luck to receive a wonderful array of cosmetic dental services for a fraction of the cost. Dental students have to have a certain amount of hands-on practice hours for their education. Under the supervision of the dental instructor (who is always close by), you can have practically any dental work preformed for almost nothing. An added bonus, since students are schooled in the latest technology, is that your service is going to be state of the art. Here are some common dental procedures:

> **FILLINGS:** Removing the amalgam (mercury) fillings and substituting composite (plastic and ceramic) or porcelain filling will give you an all-white wide-open yawn/laugh instead of a mouth like the inside of an ironworker. Besides making

you look prettier when your teeth are showing, removing the amalgam fillings may help your general health, as evidence is leaning towards mercury fillings releasing considerable amounts of neurotoxic mercury. The mercury can cause a wide range of illnesses such as allergies, headaches, fatigue syndromes, and even skin conditions. Just the cosmetic benefits alone of a crisp white smile, inside and out, are worth the decision to "get the lead out!"

BRACES: While your schoolmates may have worn braces as a child, there are now more pleasant treatment options for adults. Realignment may take longer as an adult, but huge advances have been made since the tin grins of the past— the new braces are almost invisible to the eye. Applied either to the back of the teeth for complete secrecy, or with the new invisible line at the front of the teeth, you now do not have to "brace" yourself for the treatment. More and more adults are fixing the smile that they maybe wanted to, but could not afford to, growing up. Straight teeth are as close as a few visits from the dentist.

CROWNS. A crown is the traditional way to repair a broken or unsightly tooth. It involves grinding the tooth down to a peg and fitting a replica over the top. Crowns are made to last for years—up to thirty, with continued daily care.

BRIDGES: Sometimes permanent teeth need to be replaced. You can lose a tooth through dental decay or in accidents. The dentist will create what is known as a bridge. It entails creating manufactured teeth to go over the missing teeth. It covers two teeth, which support the bridge of the missing tooth or teeth.

BONDING: A tooth-colored material is applied to an existing tooth as an alternative to crowning. The tooth is prepared to allow a porcelain inlay to be attached to the front of the tooth. Bonding is an easy fix to fill in gaps between widely spaced front and other teeth. It only lasts about five years.

VENEERS: Veneer is a popular solution for badly discolored or misshapen teeth. A very thin layer of porcelain, rather like a false fingernail, is bonded to the tooth. It fits the front side of the tooth and is another option to bonding or shaping of the tooth. Veneers are very popular because they are so thin and somewhat resistant to staining.

IMPLANTS: Titanium screw implants have revolutionized the replacement of lost teeth so that no one needs to worry about wearing dentures—if the need arises. Advanced surgical procedures allow the implant of a titanium screw into the bone of the jaw to allow a permanent replacement tooth to be inserted. Implants, while not inexpensive, last a lifetime.

BLEACHING: While all of the other services require a dentist to perform, bleaching the teeth can be done at the dental office or at home. The professional bleaching versions are laser tooth whitening and dental tray systems.

LASER: Laser is the most expensive method by far. The treatment consists of a nondamaging hydrogen peroxide–based gel applied to the teeth, then a laser is used to activate the gel and initiate the whitening process. The treatment takes about one hour and will lighten your teeth by up to six shades. Expect some sensitivity to the mouth for a couple of days. The good part is your teeth are light and bright in only one hour. The downside is the cost, from $1,000 upward, and the possible teeth and gum sensitivity.

DENTAL TRAY: With the dental tray lightening treatment, the dentist creates custom-made trays (from rubber molds) for your upper and lower teeth. At home, you fill the trays with a bleaching solution (hydrogen peroxide in various percentages, depending on the lightening desired) and insert the trays daily for the next two weeks. It is recommended that you sleep with the trays on, as you cannot drink or eat with the trays in place. The gel coats the teeth and, over the course of time, lightens the teeth. The cost averages $400 and up. The good part about the dental tray treatment is that it is less aggressive to the surrounding gums that the laser lightening. Also, you have control over when you will wear the trays and for how long. Since teeth lightening is not a permanent thing, by having the trays already made, when you want to lighten them up a bit, you just put the trays in for a few nights to bring back the brightness. The laser treatment, on the other hand, requires another costly session to return to light.

AT-HOME TEETH WHITENING TREATMENTS

Once again, thanks to technological advancements, treatments that used to be doctor-only sessions now can be done at home on your own house call—without spending thousands of dollars.

RAZZLE DAZZLE

The effects of teeth whitening methods are not permanent. Heavily pigmented foods, coffee, tea, cigarettes, and red wine all will stain teeth over time. Some suggestions are to drink white wine instead of red; substitute cappuccino for espresso; and try grapefruit juice instead of grape or cranberry. And, of course, if you smoke, whiter teeth are just one of the many health benefits you'll experience if you quit. When you notice that your teeth are not as bright as they once were, reapply your lightening method to help return the teeth to their beautiful best.

The market is full of more affordable options to have the light bright smile that you have always wanted. Here are a few of the most popular and more affordable ones.

Tray Systems

There are two kinds of tray bleaching systems that you can use at home. One is custom-made and the other is what is known as a "boil and bite" system.

Custom-Made Versions

You can buy the custom-made tray version in a kit. Inside are products that you use to create a molding of your upper and lower teeth. You mail your teeth molds to the dental lab instructed in the kit. After your custom-made trays are completed, they are mailed back to you, along with some teeth whitening gel to use with the molds. You wear the trays for a few hours a day, or overnight like the professional dental treatment. The concentration of the whitening gel is about what a dental office will give you, as this kit is more like the dental version. The cost of this version varies, but it averages about $100 for the first lightening round; the only other cost will be reordering the whitening gel for ongoing maintenance. The reorder gels are about $10 to $15 per tube.

Boil and Bite

The boil and bite type of at-home bleaching system comes with a thermoform tray that you soften by placing in boiling water and then mold to your teeth as instructed. After you have your completed trays, you put the whitening gel into the tray and follow the directions for wearing. Boil and bite tray systems are not as exact as the custom-made version but can produce a lighter and brighter smile with continued use. The cost is about $40 for the kit, and gel refills are about $6 to $8 per tube.

Gels

A new addition to the teeth lightening market is tooth gel. No need for trays, you simply apply the gel directly on the teeth and allow to stay in place for the prescribed period of time before rinsing. The cost for the gel product is about $14 for a two-week supply.

Strips

Teeth whitening strips are very popular in the marketplace as they allow you to simply put a peroxide-based gel strip right on the area that you want to lighten. You can apply one strip to your upper teeth and another strip to the lower teeth. Leave them in place for about thirty minutes. Most kits recommend that you use them two times a week for thirty minutes each session. The cost for the strip systems runs between $25 and $40 for ten applications.

Toothpastes

Especially designed whitening toothpastes (which are higher in concentration that the regular whitening toothpastes on the shelves) are available from specialty retailers as well as catalogs. Whitening toothpastes have special chemical or polishing agents that provide additional stain removal, as well as various percentages of whitening agents. It is a good idea to check with your dentist about these toothpastes, as they could be too strong for your tooth enamel with continued use.

Now more than ever it is possible to have the smile that you have always wanted. And with all of the methods available, it is enough to put a smile on every Thrifty Girl's face!

Chapter Twenty-one

Thirty Thrifty Tips for Your Beautiful Body

" Our bodies are our gardens—
our wills are our gardeners. "
—WILLIAM SHAKESPEARE

1. Self-tanning products applied to the hands, feet, and legs make them look younger, and manicures and pedicures make them look prettier.

2. Don't be fooled into thinking that being under an umbrella or a tree while out in the sun will give you enough sun protection. An umbrella eliminates only part of the ultraviolet rays. You need the same amount of sun protection as if you were sitting directly in the sun.

3. Sunshine accessories such as a hat and oh so chic sunglasses will protect you while you sashay your way to the pool or beach, as well as give you glamour galore.

4. The nape of the neck is one of the most sensual beauty zones. You may not notice it, but others certainly do. Be sure to hydrate and add sun protection to this very beautiful area.

5. Show off toned and self-tanned legs with a body moisturizer that contains shimmering ingredients such as gold or bronze flecks. Blend the product along the shin bone to give a sexy sheen and create the illusion of slimmer legs.

6. Make your own at-home version of gam glam by mixing a bit of hair shine product with a little bit of shimmery face powder and apply to legs.

7. If evening plans call for an outfit with a little shoulder, back, or décolleté action happening, sweep a large powder brush with a little glimmer powder across the areas. As you move, the glimmery powder will create little starlike twinkles—making you the star.

8. Eighty degrees is the best water temperature for bathing or showering. Any warmer, and the water will drain your energy. Any colder, and your heart may begin to race. Plus,

overly warm water removes too much of the skin's natural body oils, which keep the body moisturized.

9. When washing your hands, slow down and take your time. To get the hands truly clean, you have to wash for about thirty seconds—about the time it takes to sing "Happy Birthday." Anything less, and they are most likely not clean.

10. If your ankles tend to swell from walking or warm weather, soak your feet in a bowl of warm water and four tablespoons of Epsom salts. This will ease the swelling and soothe tired feet. You can return telephone calls or read your mail, all the while depuffing your feet.

11. To whiten yellowed fingernails or toenails, soak the nails in white vinegar for ten minutes. Rinse dry and apply cuticle cream. If the stain is stubborn, mix 2 tablespoons of household bleach and ½ cup of warm water. Place nails in mixture for fifteen minutes. Be sure to rinse well, and slather on the moisturizing cream afterwards.

12. Barefoot it. Any chance that you get to kick off your shoes and go bare, go for it. Walking along a sandy beach or on a grassy patch of lawn feels wonderful and is good for your sole—and your soul.

13. A great backup plan for broken-out backs is to mix together 2 tablespoons of apple cider vinegar with 1 cup of warm water. Soak a washcloth in the mixture and gently cleanse the entire back area. Allow to dry. Do not rinse. This treatment will rid the back area of bacteria and excess dead skin cells—both of which could be causing the breakouts. Apply this treatment once or twice a week until the blemishes have banished.

14. For body breakouts, a detoxifying bath of one cup of aloe vera juice mixed in a tub of very warm water can work wonders to help clear the breakouts. Soak the entire body up to the neck in the solution for ten minutes. Then take a washcloth and pour some aloe vera juice onto the cloth until it is saturated. Gently cleanse the affected areas with the cloth. Immerse your skin once again in the tub to rinse and pat dry.

15. If hot weather makes you sticky, try adding a bit of baking soda or cornstarch to your body powder before applying. Baking soda or cornstarch absorbs excess moisture as well as odor. This is great for underarms, if your deodorant has a tendency to stain or discolor clothing. Baby products often contain these ingredients, if you want a ready-to-go product. Check them out in the baby care aisle.

16. To help you sleep at night, open the curtains as soon as you get up. Bright natural sunlight early in the day enhances the body's internal rhythms and helps you sleep better at night.

17. Tuck a lavender sachet under your pillow before leaving for the day. When you are ready for bed, your entire bed will smell wonderful and relaxing.

18. To check to see if your breath is less than fresh, lick your freshly washed palm and smell it while it's still wet. If it is, you can grab a mint ASAP. Covering your mouth with your hand and breathing into it doesn't work—but the wet palm never fails.

19. Applying a layer of top coat to your manicure every day will allow your manicure to last all week. Plus, the additional layers help protect the nails from peeling or breaking.

20. For a spa treatment while doing household chores, slather your hands with hand cream before putting on your rubber gloves. The gloves will keep the hands warm and allow the cream to penetrate. For an added bonus, if your chores require working in warm water, the hand spa treatment will work even better.

21. Before putting on sandals, give the feet a little spritz of cologne. It will instantly cool the feet as well as allow a little fragrance to waft as you walk.

22. To keep nail polish from bubbling up on the nails, do not shake the polish bottle. Instead, turn the bottle upside down and gently roll the bottle side to side in the palms of your hand.

23. If the shape of your toenails is square, the colors that look the most classic are the darker shades. If your toenails are rounder in shape, the most elegant colors to wear are reds and pinks.

24. Nails also need protection from the sun. Use a top coat enriched with UVA and UVB filters. This will also help keep the color looking fresh and discoloring less.

25. To keep from undoing your 'do while bathing, run a little cold water in the tub or shower before you turn on the hot. This will lessen the steam that causes the hair to go flat.

26. For the price of two tea bags, you can have a spa experience. As the bathtub is filling with water, tie the two tea bags underneath the faucet so that the water runs through the bag. The water will be wonderfully scented and filled with skin-loving antioxidants. As you lie back, put the tea bags over your closed eyes to relieve and refresh your eyes.

27. As you wash your delicates such as undergarments and hosiery, add a drop or two of your signature fragrance to the rinse water. You will take your special fragrance with you in a wonderfully understated way.

28. Practice makes perfect—for pictures, that is. Practice posing for photographs in front a mirror. Look at your smile. How do your eyes look? Do you look like you're posed, or do you look natural? Put one of your feet and legs slightly forward and angle the body for the most flattering picture.

29. If you suffer from dry itchy skin and scalp, invest in a room humidifier. You can turn it on while you sleep and ease the dry, itchy skin. Plus, moist air, especially in the winter months, will make breathing easier.

30. Glamour girls are always ready for the getaway. Keep a waterproof toilette bag packed with travel sizes of all of your can't-live-without products. That way, you will be ready to seize the day—any day of the week!

PART 5

THE
THRIFTY
GIRL'S
GUIDE TO
GLAMOROUS
FASHION

One of the areas where it's hardest to be thrifty while still looking glamorous is your closet. This section will teach you how to avoid shopping "misses," and how to shop on a budget—but still be a total hit.

Chapter Twenty-two

Chic Physique

❝ Cultivate your curves—they may be dangerous but they won't be avoided. ❞

—MAE WEST

Have you ever wondered why that great-looking pair of jeans fit your friend like a glove, yet missed the mark completely when you tried them on—even when you're the same size? Or how about the oh so chic dress that your ordered from the catalog that just hung like it was still on the hanger when you tried it on? The answer to these and more questions on why sometimes it fits and sometimes it doesn't, and how come one outfit makes you feel gorgeous while another one makes you feel frumpy is—body shape.

If you are not dressing for your body shape, you are missing out on the true secret to looking fabulous—all of the time—not just getting lucky now and then.

Educating yourself about your body shape allows you to always purchase and wear clothing that keeps you on the "divine dressing" list.

THE BODY SILHOUETTE

Research indicates that women's figures today are slowing becoming less shapely and curvy compared to previous generations. The 1950s were, the decade of the voluptuous hourglass figure, such as that of Marilyn Monroe (37-23-36). In the 1960s, Twiggy was the extreme opposite of the curvy woman, with stats of 32-22-32. The supermodels of the 1980s and '90s averaged measurements of 33-23-34, and today's statistical icon varies, depending on who is on the red carpet—or which diet the latest celebrity is on.

THE SHAPE OF THINGS TO COME

If you want to smooth out extra lumps and bumps to create a slimmer silhouette, try a body shaper. Unlike the old-fashioned constricting girdle, a body shaper simply creates a smoother look at the waist, hips, thighs, and bum by holding everything firm. Shapers come in several lengths; some end at the thigh, some at the knee, and some go all the way to the capri length—which is perfect for close-fitting pants.

The fact is that, over time, bodies change. The hips become bigger, waists become thicker, and busts become smaller. Some female body shapes become more athletic, creating fewer curves but more defined muscles. And while all of this contributes to the ever-changing body shape phenomenon, there are still essentially just five body shapes. One of these body shape categories you can call your very own.

Pear

Also known as A framed or triangle-shaped, pear shapes tend to be full and wide at the bottom and narrow and slim at the top. The top half features a small bust, defined waist, and smaller shoulders. The lower half has thicker hips, thighs, and buttocks. Pears tend to put on weight in the saddlebag area first. Goldie Hawn and Meryl Streep are good examples of slender pear shapes.

Pears: What to Wear

The clothing goal for pear-shaped bodies is to balance the shape, focusing on widening the shoulders. Wearing lighter colors, wide lapels, and shoulder pads will create body harmony and create a balanced look.

- Straight skirts should be tapered toward the hemline to avoid a square-body look.
- Pants should be made of flowing fabrics and drape loosely around the hips.
- Shoulder pads are your best dressing friend.
- Blouses should not end where your bottom does—this will accentuate the area that you are tying to minimize.
- Create emphasis on the upper body with semi-fitting and tailored tops.
- Handbags should be worn above the hip area to avoid drawing attention to the hips.
- Cowl necks, square necklines, and interesting collars will help broaden the shoulder area.
- Accessories such as scarves that drape around the neck (but do not extend to the waist) and bulky ethnic jewelry are eye-catching and very flattering to pear shapes.
- Keep heel height and style simple, as platforms and chunky heels weigh the shape down.

Cone

Also known as the inverted triangle shape, or T shaped, cone shapes have a broad shoulder and bust over a narrow hip and waist. Thighs are slim and buttocks are flat, while the legs and arms are long, muscular, and shapely. Cone shapes carry most of their weight in their shoulders, busts, and backs. Many athletic women are cone-shaped. Jamie Lee Curtis is a good example of a cone shape.

Cones: What to Wear

To balance the cone shape, visually widen the hips and upper legs. Choosing skirts and wider-leg pants will add fullness where you want it.

- High-set sleeves visually narrow wide shoulders.
- Patch pockets will create interest and soften the look of broader shoulders.
- Flared skirts will add shape to the legs to balance with the top.
- Flared-leg pants are great for cone shapes.
- Low-slung belts help add a bit of bulk to the hips as well as interest, with a great belt.
- Dusters and "lab" coats ensembles are good to elongate cone shapes.
- Shoulder pads—if used at all—should be minimum size.
- Delicate knit sweaters are great to show off the shoulders.
- Sexy high heels were made for this body shape. If you got it, flaunt it.

Rectangle

Also known as the slender shape or H shape, rectangle shapes resemble a rectangle, as they are straight up and down, front and back, with few to no curves. The upper and lower are proportionate; however, there is little to no waist on rectangle shapes. The main assets of rectangle shapes are that the bust is longer, and the arms and legs are long and slender. Mary-Kate and Ashley Olsen have rectangle shapes.

Rectangles: What to Wear

The goal is to create the illusion of a smaller, shapelier waist. A bloused top with a flared skirt, or a chemise-style dress, are figure flattering styles.

- Avoid belts, as they will accentuate the thickness of the waist.
- Dresses that fit loose in the midsection are a good selection.
- A shirtdress-type style will look smart.
- Try V-necklines, which are slenderizing and elongate the neck.
- Any neckline that falls below the collarbone will help create a longer-looking neck.
- Longer jackets with shorter skirts help to visually lengthen the upper torso.
- Dropped-waist skirts elongate the upper torso and will help slenderize.
- Avoid very gathered or heavily pleated fabric at the waist.
- Straight, long-tailored shirts paired with a longer tunic top will create a great look.
- Semifitted pants or jeans under a longer-length top will accentuate the positive aspects of your shape.
- Any shoes that draw attention to the legs are a go.

Apple

Also known as the round or the O shape, apple shapes are rounder, carrying most of the weight in the midsection. Apple shapes are characterized by an ample neck, generous bust, wider rib cage, round back, generous middle, with narrow hips and shapely legs. Kate Winslet is a good example of a slender apple shape.

The dressing goal for apples is create a longer, leaner torso while adding emphasis to the shapely legs.

- Avoid fitted tops that will accentuate a larger middle.
- Steer away from bulky or gathered skirts.
- A more tailored fit will flatter your best asset—your legs.
- Avoid wide belts that divide your body in half.
- Narrow belts that blend with the colors being worn will create the illusion of a waist.
- Handbags should hit at the hip level and lower.
- V-necklines and elongated necklines will help slenderize the neck.
- Collars and lapels should be narrow and small so as not draw attention to the wider top area.
- Longer tunics help hide a more generous middle and draw the attention down to the legs.
- Shoulder pads are not recommended, as they add weight where you do not need it.
- Double-breasted anything should be not worn, as it adds bulk.
- Keep shoes to the classic pump or low heels.

Hourglass

Also known as the figure 8 and the Eve shape, the hourglass shape is the most balanced of all shapes. The frame features the same width of shoulder to hips with a very well-defined waist in between.

EMPTY YOUR POCKETS

Carrying items in pockets adds visual weight to your hips and thighs. Instead, why not put everything in a flattering and stylish handbag?

Curvy best describes the hourglass shape. The bust, hips, thighs, tummy, and buttocks are on the rounded side. Halle Berry is an example of an hourglass shape.

Hourglass: What to Wear

The goal here is to emphasize the waist by selecting garments that fit the body and call attention to the waist, such as shirtwaist styles, and set-in waist with fitted tops and flared skirts.

- Oversize and baggy styles will hide what nature gave you.
- Draw attention to the waist with waistbands, belts, and wrap tops that tie at the waist.
- Avoid clothing that is too fitted, as it will not look as expensive but rather cheap.
- Semifitted is the most slimming for this shape.
- A softly fitted sweater can show off the curves.
- Avoid too much bulk to the top or the bottom, as it will hide the figure.
- High heels and middle heels create height and a bit of drama for this perfect shape.

BODY ISSUES

Now that you have determined your body shape, you may be saying to yourself, "I think that I have it down, but I also have other figure issues," such as wanting to look taller, shorter, make the bust look bigger or smaller, etc. Instead of spending a million on plastic surgery, follow this guide to help you with any individual figure concerns. Simply use the tips to "fake" your body shape outline and create your own personal chic physique.

LOOK TALLER: Create length by line verticals such as buttons on the top; jackets with piping going down the front;

dressing from head to toe in one color (known as mono-chromatic dressing); blending clothing color with stocking and shoe color. Stay away from horizontal elements that break up the line, creating a "cut in half" look.

LOOK SHORTER: Horizontal elements are great to shorten the torso. Choose contrasting colors such as a bright color jacket with a neutral skirt or pants; patterns and prints of medium to large scale help scale down height. Stay away from one-color dressing and patterns and prints that are too small and delicate.

SHORTEN A LONG NECK: Turtlenecks, cowl necks, and standup-neck collars are easy ways to hide a longer neck. Scarves and necklaces will break up the lines. Stay away from V-necklines as they add length; long dangling earrings will also add extra length.

ADD LENGTH TO THE NECK: V-necklines and open collars create length where little exists; as does a shawl or roll-neck necklines. Stay away from: scarves, necklaces, pins, and anything that keeps the eye on the neck area.

SCALE DOWN BROAD SHOULDERS: Raglan, dolman, and flowing sleeves draw attention to the arms and away from the shoulders. V-necklines add emphasis to the neck and create a middle-of-the-body focal point, like a scarf or an interesting longer necklace does. Stay away from ruffled collars, shoulder pads, and design details like epaulets and yokes on the shoulders.

BROADEN SHOULDERS: Add shoulder pads to everything. Bateau and boat-neck lines are flattering. Choose horizontal patterns for jackets or blouse tops. Stay away from halter tops; dolman and raglan sleeves will make the shoulders look smaller.

MINIMIZE FULL BUST: V-necklines are good to create a narrowing line downward; shawls and other interesting collars draw attention up to the face and away from the bust. Both necklaces and earrings, as well as scarves, will capture the eye's attention. Stay away from ruffles, bows, tube tops, and breast pocket details, horizontal stripes and wide belts almost under the breast.

CREATE A FULLER BUST: Layers are a great way to create fullness; shorter jackets, vest, and bolero-style tops are great ways to add a little where there isn't, and keeping tops bright and lighter than the bottoms will create the illusion of more. Stay away from tops that are too tight and clingy or low cut, as well as styles such as an empire waist.

SHORTEN A LONG WAIST: Choose tops with stripes. Pocket details are good, and empire waist styles help shorten the image. Wear wider belts that are in the same color as your skirt or pants. Stay away from long jackets or blouses over short skirts or cropped pants. Avoid narrow or hip-length belts.

LENGTHEN A SHORT WAIST: Drop-waist dresses and no-waist styles are good for this figure. Longer jackets or overblouses will lengthen, and keeping the color of the belt matching the top color as opposed to matching the pants or skirt will create a longer silhouette. Stay away from wide belts; short jackets or empire styles will also shorten the torso.

THIN A THICK WAIST: Keep belts on the narrow side and make the belt buckle the focus point. Free-flowing garments and tunic tops hide what you do not want noticed. Stay away from any color changing around the waist such as belt color or scarf color, if the scarf ends at the waist area.

LESSEN THE TUMMY: Keep the eye upward toward the neckline with great jewelry and earrings. Shoulder lines and detail are good for creating a thinner tummy; longer tops that are hip length and longer will carry the eye elsewhere. Stay away from gathered, full skirts; pleats on pants or skirt fronts; anything shiny or bulky will add bulk where you do not want or need it.

DECREASING THE HIPS: Keep the attention on the top half of the body—shoulder and neck details are wonderful ways to draw the eyes up. Choose straight, fuller leg pants and keep the colors on the bottom half neutral and dark, while adding colors to the top part of the body. Stay away from anything that draws attention to the hip area. Avoid clothing that is too fitted, opt instead for semi-fitted. Plaids, patterns, and stripes are not good for the bottom half of the body; and strappy sandals or ankle straps on shoes create a larger hip, leg, and foot.

CREATE A HIP: Peplum jackets are great to add a little girth to the hip. Boxy jackets with full skirts add some inches and longer blouses worn outside a skirt or pants belted with a middle-size belt create a hip line. Stay away from knits of any kind—pants, skirts, or dresses will emphasis the lack of bum, and clothes that cling or sag in the seat are not flattering.

ELONGATE LEGS: Keep the hemlines on pants just a bit longer, without going too long. Choose hosiery to match the hem and shoe for the longest leg look. Vertical details like pinstripes, pleats, and buttons in a vertical line will create a longer length in general to the body. Stay away from capri pants or styles that are horizontal, which will shorten the body and the legs.

LESSEN LONG LEGS: Choose jackets and tops that end past the hip or thigh and keep skirt lengths below the knee or mid-calf. Stay away from a one-color look on bottoms, hosiery, and shoes. High-waist skirts or pants will elongate the look of the legs rather than lessening.

SLENDERIZE ARMS: Loosely fitted sleeves such as dolman or kimono will flatter your arms, shoulder pads in small to medium size will create a cleaner line, and shoulder details on tops will draw the eye upward and away from the arms. Sleeves that can be pushed up add a slimming silhouette. Stay away from clinging or tight fabrics, and short or cap sleeves will add rather than subtract—don't even think about sleeveless.

DISGUISE THIN, LONGER ARMS: Free-flowing sleeves of fabric are good choices. Long sleeves with French cuffs or other interesting cuff detail are also an option. Stay away from tight sleeves, pushed-up sleeves, and sleeveless or strapless tops.

This chapter covers a lot of dressing details. But as Coco Chanel so eloquently stated, "Beauty is in the details." Once you have determined your personal chic physique details and know what makes you look great—and not so great—you are now ready to make *The Thrifty Girl's Guide to Glamour* Pledge: that you will only dress in what makes you look and feel your beautiful best from this day forward. Let your first impression last.

Chapter Twenty-three

Taking Fashion
Personally

" Fashion can be bought; but style
you must possess. "
—EDNA WOOLMAN CHASE

How many times have you opened the closet door and stared at a closet full of clothes, and yet you feel as if you have nothing to wear? Is your style image one that you want to project, or are bored with your look? Do you find yourself dressing for others instead of for you? If you have answered yes to any of these questions, perhaps you need to start taking your fashion personally.

YOUR SIGNATURE STYLE

The first step to finding your fashion personality is defining who you are when it comes to style. This is a critical step that most women overlook. Instead, many of us go with this trend or follow that mood, buy what is in the magazines or on TV, or wear what the salesclerk tells us looks good. Taking your fashion personally does not start by shopping at a store. It cannot be forced when you have a dressing deadline like a wedding, a big meeting, or an important luncheon. It starts with a pencil and paper, and a few dressing memories.

CLIP IT IN THE BUD

Clip out photos of looks you like from catalogs and magazines that most closely match your style. This will help you to be a smart shopper before you even leave the house.

Take a minute and think about your absolute favorite outfit. Think about the one outfit that you often want to wear on a special occasion, a date, a business function, or whatever the occasion may be. Once you have determined your very best feel-good, look-fabulous outfit, jot it down.

Ask yourself these questions, and record your answers.

1. Why do you like that outfit?

   ■ Is it the cut of the garment?
   ■ Is it the color?
   ■ Is it that you feel beautiful in it?
   ■ Is the one that you get the most compliments on?

2. Write down three adjectives to describe how you feel in it.

   ■ Perhaps it makes you feel powerful, pretty, sensual, totally together. Whatever. Just write down three adjectives to describe how it makes you feel.

The outfit you like best will provide great insight into your style. Why? If you feel powerful or very professional, then you enjoy the corporate image. If you like that you get a lot of compliments, then you probably bask in the limelight. If comfort is the main consideration, then dressing is something you just *have* to do. If you say it makes you feel pretty or sensual, then that is the look that most fits your fashion personality.

THRIFTY TIP

While it is always a refreshing change to buy an outfit that you like, yet it does not fit into your usual style profile, you should recognize that your style is just that—your style. Buying something that is dramatically different from your usual style may result in a purchase that never sees the world outside your closet.

There are four distinctly different dressing styles. They are Classic Sophisticate; Dramatic Trendsetter; Natural Chic; and Feminine Romantic.

CLASSIC SOPHISTICATE

This fashion personality is the epitome of style and grace. Classic Sophisticates want timeless pieces. They prefer rich fabrics, superb tailoring, and tasteful, expensive jewelry and accessories. They can pull something from their wardrobe that they bought five years ago and still be in style. Classic Sophisticates always look pulled together from head to toe—the bag, the shoes, the jewelry, all compliment the outfit outstandingly. The clothes are simple and elegant. This personality is fashionable, but never faddish or severe. *Tailored* is the word of the day. However, she can sometimes look too safe and too controlled. She may want to loosen up her look with a few unexpected fashion touches.

Some Classic Sophisticate preferences include:

- Plain fabrics, soft florals, impressionistic watercolor prints, houndstooth and herringbone prints, muted glen plaids
- Medium to lightweight fabrics like fine wools, silks, jerseys, cashmere, suede, gabardine
- Matte-finish fabrics preferred to those with high luster for evening
- Expensive-looking jewelry, even if it is costume
- Tailored shoulder bags, satchels, and envelope styles
- Simple pumps with low to medium heels, spectator pumps, and slingbacks
- Elegant leather or skin belts with simple buckles
- Finely textured hosiery in sheer colors
- Soft and sleek hair
- Makeup perfectly understated; overall balance of eyes, cheeks, and lips, in medium intensity colors. A Classic Sophisticate woman avoids looking overdone, but this can sometimes lead to a look that is too safe and conservative. She may want to experiment with brighter, more intense makeup colors, for a classic style that is all her own.

Famous Classic Sophisticates are Grace Kelly, Coco Chanel, Renee Zellweger, Ivana Trump, Maria Shriver, and Vanessa Williams.

DRAMATIC TRENDSETTER

This fashion personality is a fashion-forward person. By the time everyone else is starting to follow a certain trend, the dramatic trendsetter is already bored and onto something else. She loves clothes. This style enjoys bold, bright colors, one-of-a-kind jewelry pieces, and out-of-the-ordinary fashion looks. She wears high fashion comfortably, and for her, style is an overriding concern.

Although the Dramatic Trendsetter woman can wear more tailored clothing during the day, at night she typically chooses more of an extreme and exotic look. High fashion is designed for a Dramatic Trendsetter personality, but in the workplace she may have to downplay her drama. A good strategy for her is to buy simple clothing with more classic lines that she can accessorize with varying degrees of drama depending on the occasion. This way she can maximize every outfit.

Some Dramatic Trendsetter preferences are:

- Solid colors or boldly printed fabrics that are usually abstract or geometric in form
- Textures that vary from firm weaves that tailor or drape well, such as crepe, broadcloth, gabardine, and worsted to soft jersey
- For evening, lustrous fabrics like satin, heavy brocade, and lamé
- Accessories that vary from the bold plan and are large, elaborate, ornate, and lavish
- One-of-a-kind jewelry pieces, bright costume jewelry, rhinestones, bold geometric shapes, many chains and bracelets

- Oversize handbags in unstructured shapes and a variety of skins and leather textures
- A wide variety of shoes in different colors and styles to match many outfits, and at least two pairs of boots
- A variety of large and small belts with interesting buckles and chains
- Colorful, textured hosiery stashed in a drawer for a wild dressing day
- Super-sleek or tousled hair
- The latest, most extreme makeup looks; never skimps on makeup, instinctively playing up her best features. Her style is striking but could at times, be a little over-the-top. It is important that the Dramatic Trendsetter strive for a balanced, harmonious look, to keep from appearing overdone.

Famous Drama Trendsetters include Charlize Theron, Gwen Stefani, Whoopi Goldberg, Shirley MacLaine, and of course, the Queen of Dramatic Trendsetting—Cher.

NATURAL CHIC

The difference between a Natural Chic and a Dramatic Trendsetter is that that Natural Chic goes completely for comfort while a Dramatic Trendsetter will wear it even if it hurts! A Natural Chic fashion personality likes a fresh, clean look and sports understated colors. Natural Chic dressers are typically relaxed, casual people, and this is apparent in the style of their clothing. Sporty or traditional separates are the Natural Chic woman's favorite look, and comfort is key. Even the formalwear will be very simple in line but made of beautiful fabrics.

The Natural Chic uses restraint in her clothing design and accessories, but sometimes she looks underdressed. Slightly larger or bolder accessories will give her a more polished, up-to-the-minute look.

Some Natural Chic preferences are:

- Solid fabrics
- Plaids, checks, stripes, and all-over prints
- Uneven or rough textures, like tweed, rough linen, raw silk, or hand-knitted textures, and plain-surfaced fabric jersey knits or gabardine
- Simple jewelry in gold and sliver, colored stones, and no-nonsense watches
- Traditional or soft shoulder bags and clutches
- Low-heeled pumps and boots, penny loafers, and athletic shoes
- Simple, casual-looking belts worn with separates
- Fun socks worn with casual shoes and sheer or lightly textured hosiery
- An easy-to-care-for hairstyle
- An "all-American" look. Her makeup is always clean and fresh, but can sometimes look underdone. She may want to try experimenting with more makeup, and brighter shades of lipstick.

Some well-known Natural Chic fashion personalities are Sandra Bullock, Jennifer Garner, Katie Holmes, Katie Couric, and Cindy Crawford.

FEMININE ROMANTIC

The Feminine Romantic is the epitome of femininity and sex appeal, and she places femininity over chic every time. She wears soft, flowing dresses and lightly tailored suites with silky blouses, scarves, and soft sweaters. She will treasure cameos, lockets, and antique-looking pieces. A romantic must be careful to not overdo the ruffles and lace in the workplace, or to choose working styles that look "little girlish." Soft suits and feminine accessories will satisfy her romantic nature yet look professional.

Feminine Romantic preferences include:

- Medium to light-weight fabrics like fine silk, crepe, jersey, plain knits, fine cotton, soft woolens, and cashmere
- For prints, soft blended florals, polka dots, dotted swiss, eyelet, embroidery, and soft plaids
- Formal fabrics of velvet, lace, chiffon or voile; fake fur and feather
- Jewelry that is dainty in detail but lavish in effect, added to the cameos, and antique pieces perhaps with some nice costume pearls; might wear several jewelry pieces at a time
- Handbags that are small and have feminine touches in design
- High strapping pumps and flats with buckles and bows
- Thin delicate belts or chains, attractive buckles or wide colorful sashes
- Sheer and finely textured hosiery
- Soft and full hair
- The picture of soft femininity; loves a delicate Victorian look with pale, subdued makeup. She should be careful of appearing too delicate in the workplace by wearing darker, more intense colors. She is attracted to lip glosses, but may want to add a few lipsticks for a more professional makeup look.

Feminine Romantic examples include Sophia Loren, Jane Seymour, Halle Berry, Catherine Zeta-Jones, and Jennifer Lopez.

Your fashion personality is your visible calling card. In order to have a totally put-together look that reflects who you are, the style theme needs to be carried from head to toe. Think about it. Have you ever seen a Feminine Romantic personality wearing lace only to confuse the look with geometric earrings? Or what about a totally one-of-a-kind Dramatic Trendsetter outfit with sensible shoes? The look is incomplete and out of whack. A true sense of style can be heard in the compliment "I saw an outfit today, and it would be perfect for you." That means that you are taking fashion personally and have created a sense of style that is recognizable to others.

BALANCING BUDGET AND STYLE

Sometimes budget dictates style. But if money were no object, how would you dress to fit your fashion personality? When you look at fashion magazines, which styles are you most often drawn to? Or if you are not at your ideal weight, would being the perfect weight change your clothing style at all?

STYLE SLEUTH

If you are still on the fence as to fashion personality, why not plan a shopping spree with a friend? Here's the catch: bring absolutely no money. This spree is for fact-finding only. While window-shopping, discover clothing and accessories that enhance who you are. Once you have assembled a couple of perfect outfits for you, look at them very closely—you will discover your true fashion personality.

You may be drawn to more than one clothing style, just as a Classic Sophisticate may choose more Dramatic Trendsetter clothing for the weekends, or slip on a more Natural Chic look with children's activities. However, there is usually one particular style that most closely matches your fashion personality. And once it is identified, it is easer to manage a wardrobe and manage your entire look, to say nothing about being able to finally find something to wear in your closet!

Chapter Twenty-four

Coming Out of the Closet

" No more wire hangers . . . ever! "

—FAYE DUNAWAY AS JOAN CRAWFORD,
IN *MOMMY DEAREST*

Just thinking about the words *closet organizing*, let alone saying them out loud, is enough to send shivers up many a girl's spine. Conquering the closet clutter, clothes, and chaos once and for all but is a grand and wonderful thing, the "getting there" part is enough to make you want to close the door, and put a "do not disturb" sign on the knob. Better yet, why not move and give your closet your new forwarding address!

Clothes can hang around for years, if not decades. Why can't clothes come with expiration dates? If clothes were food, you would know when to toss them. Smooth silks would become corduroys; solid greens would turn into madras plaids. Dehydration would make dresses shrivel up three sizes.

Flashy, trendy, bright colored clothes would have a six-month usage date. Right beside the care instructions label would be a usage label: "Best used by September 22, 2008." Neutral colors and simple classic designs would be less perishable: "Best if used by May 15, 2010." You would not need a second opinion about the floral dress with the puffy sleeves, or the robin's egg blue painter pants, before giving it the boot. And if your significant other questioned why you are hauling out a garbage bag or two of clothing, you would simply say, "Look right here, honey, they all say use before June 23, 2006." No guilt would be involved. It is simply a matter of an expiration date—when the date arrives, out it goes.

But it is hard to get rid of clothes as so far the fashion industry has given us no inside tags to alert us when they are past their prime. And while we know in our fashion-sense mind that an item has become a liability instead of an asset, somehow it lingers well past its wearable prime. After all, it is in perfectly good shape. No rips, no tears, no stains. It might come back in style, after all, like they say: "Everything old is new again"—right?

It is time to come out of the closet and create a haven for your fashion personality—making dressing a daily pleasure, instead of a chore, day in and day out. Let's get started.

SEVEN STEPS TO CLOSET HEAVEN

Warning: This is a hard and sometimes painful process, but you have to remove all of the pieces that you have never felt right in. If they don't match your fashion personality, they are not doing you any good. Plus, they are taking up valuable closet space.

THRIFTY TIP

Clothes whose only function is taking up valuable closet space are causing you more aggravation than good. It is probably these clothes that, when you look at them or try them on, a bad mood suddenly hits you. You are so much better off without them. Donating them to a charity will ease the guilt and allow someone else to enjoy them for real!

While overhauling your closet may seem like a totally overwhelming task, here are seven steps to get you started.

1. **Establish an Identity.** Your image tells the outside world who you are on the inside. How you look, dress, and accessorize is the window to your personality—and your fashion personality.

2. **Lifestyle Assessment.** To assess your wardrobe needs, take a look at your lifestyle in percentages. Add up your work and/or volunteer time; casual and/or sports time; and special occasion time. You need to decide the clothing that you need for each category. As a rule of thumb, work and volunteer time should make up 65 percent of your clothing; casual and sport time about 25 percent, and special occasions should account for 10 percent.

3. **Weather Wise-Up.** The climate of your environment is critical to organizing your closet. If you live in or regularly travel to an area with four distinctly different seasons, your best investment is all-season clothing that you can layer as the weather dictates.

4. **Physical Inventory:** Time to take everything out of your closet—yes, everything—and sort your clothing into four piles:

- The "where is that salesgirl *now*" pile: This will be the pile that you give away or sell at a consignment store.
- The "mend your ways" pile: This is the broken-zipper, missing-buttons, need-a-tailor pile.
- The "little weigh to go" pile: This is the pile that you cannot wear—either too big (for goodness' sake, give these away!) or the pile of clothes that are a bit too snug, but you love them.
- The "keepers" pile: This pile is most likely about 20 percent of your closet, made up of the clothes that you wear day in and day out.

5. **Take Control:** Now is the time to act on the four piles.

- Give away the giveaway pile. Remember, if you haven't worn it in a year and it fits, chances are you will not wear it again. Let someone else fall in love with it.
- Go to a tailor or get your sewing basket out and start the thread rolling.
- Put the weigh to go's in a box and label it by size. If you gain or lose weight, you'll still have these clothes. Otherwise, get rid of the guilt and get it out of the closet.
- Time to try absolutely everything on in front of a full-length mirror. Ask yourself: How does it hang? How do I feel in it? Do I really want this? Is it figure

flattering? If you have answered an honest yes to all of the questions—congratulations, it is a keeper!

- Separate all suit items from each other. Hang each jacket, skirt, and a pair of pants on a separate hanger. Suits may come married, but they do have affairs, so separate them to be able to mix and match them.

- Put all similar items together. Hang slacks, skirts, jackets, blouses, and so on together. And then further separate by color. Yes, that's right. All white blouses go with white blouses, etc.

6. **Color-edge Your Wardrobe.** Determine two colors for your wardrobe foundation. Unsure? Think about the two colors you get the most compliments on or the ones that make you feel terrific. Don't feel obligated to be safe. Don't settle for black and white if purple and lime green are your passion. Color should make you feel alive and vibrant. If your closet doesn't reflect your color preference, you may need to make some adjustments. However, from this day forward, gear your wardrobe to the colors that most accentuate your best features and just plain make you feel good.

7. **Ready, Set, Go:** Put all of the keepers back in the closet. Now is the time to go through your scarves, handbags, shoes, and jewelry to see what goes with your new look and what does not. Whether it is the shoes that kill your feet, the handbag that you need a flashlight to find anything inside of, or the brooch that weighs about two pounds, they need to be recycled back to the universe. Let someone find it as the missing link to her perfect fashion personality.

While this may seem like a huge and overwhelming project, it really will only take two or three hours to complete—about the same amount of time it takes to watch a movie. Think about how wonderful it will be not to be overwhelmed every time you open the closet door, and how happy you'll be to go shopping in your very own closet—without spending a dime!

ACCESSORIZE YOUR CLOSET

Storage and closet-organizing stores and Web sites have become very popular over the last couple of years. You can find hangers, storage bins, see-through boxes, shoe and belt holders, and more—all designed to help your closet stay neat and organized.

Choosing the same style of hangers for all of your clothing will create an eye-pleasing view of your clothes as well as keep the clothing looking neater. Hangers of various sizes and widths cause the clothing beside them to scrunch up and wrinkle more.

See-through boxes and storage bins are a great way to keep your items up close and personal yet protected and out of the way.

Shoe and belt racks are wonderful to showcase your items so that you can remember what you have!

Closet 911 Kit

Keep a grooming kit for your closet on hand to be able to handle clothing emergencies. Some must-haves for your kit include:

- **Clothes brush.** A clothing brush looks like a hairbrush with very tight bristles. It allows you to prevent dust, and other elements from clogging the garment's ability to breathe.
- **Lint brush.** A tape roller will remove lint, dust, and hair from garments.
- **Sweater shaver.** This removes the little balls or "pills" that accumulate on sweaters.
- **Instant shoeshine kit.** Like the kind that you get in a hotel room—they're great to fix a scuff or buff out a scratch on a moment's notice.

- **Sewing kit.** A compact kit with several thread colors and prethreaded needles will save you a stitch in time.
- **Hand steamer.** For quick fixes on wrinkles, a hand steamer will heat up fast and eliminate the crease in no time. Steamers are also good for freshening up ASAP.
- **Stain-removing wipes.** Portable towelettes to dab off a stain can come in very handy. You may also want to keep one in your purse or car.
- **Febreze.** It's a great product to remove smoke and odors from clothing.

While every one of us has certainly felt the need to empty our closet and start over from scratch, a Thrifty Girl knows that this is never practical. And if you take the time to revamp your closet, you'll also discover that most of the time, it's not even necessary.

Chapter Twenty-five

Diamond Dressing on a Cubic Zirconia Budget

" To sell something, tell a woman it's a bargain; tell a man it's deductible! "

—EARL WILSON

You cannot put a price on style. We have all seen clothes that cost a great deal but do not look like it. Take, for instance, the ultraexpensive torn and painted jeans costing up to $400. It is hard to believe that people actually pay serious money for pathetic, runover looking garments—but they do.

Until recently, you could almost always tell the price of a garment. But now, the garment industry is very competitive, which translates to an incredible advantage for Thrifty Girls. Slashing prices has created a clothes war of sorts on 7th Avenue. Even the designer has a difficult time identifying her own knockoffs without scrutiny. Shopping is now a dream come true. This is your knight in polished cotton!

THRIFTY TIP

CPW = Dressing Success. CPW (cost per wear) is a fabulous way to really tell what an outfit will cost you over the life of the garment. Example: You purchase a $175 ivory cashmere twin set. You sometimes wear the sweater and the shell as a set, sometimes wear just the sweater, and other times wear the shell under another topper. Either way, you wear one or both items once a week during the cooler seasons of fall and winter. Six months equals 26 weekly wearings; $175, divided by 26, equals $6.73 per wearing. And if you keep the set for three years, the cost is now only $2.24 a week—less than the price of a fancy coffee!

Or what if it is a beautiful evening suit that you can wear two times this year and once next year? It cost you $325. That's $108.33 a wearing. Is it worth it?

CZ YOUR WARDROBE

Dressing on a budget is truly a diamond in the rough. This chapter is all about "CZing" your wardrobe. Even on a cubic zirconia budget, you can still turn the heads of the rich and famous. It is time to go on a CZ shopping spree. Prepare your mind for bargains. Hold on tight to your wallet, and follow this advice:

> **STOP 1: CONSIGNMENT SHOPS.** Just a few years ago, you would not be caught dead in a used clothing store. Today, it is actually very chic to shop at a secondhand store. These hidden treasures are the secrets of the well dressed. Many don't talk about them, as they want to keep these bargains to themselves. You can pick up top designer clothes and trendy accessories that the rich may have only worn once or twice. Oddly enough, you can also find items that still have the original price tag on them. Perhaps they were bought a size too small and never felt quite right. Or maybe a jacket that is just darling was never worn because the impulse item was not "classy" enough for the club. However, it may very well be the coolest look around for a luncheon with your glamour girlfriends.

> **STOP 2: CATALOGS.** For busy woman, this fingertip method of shopping is ideal. It saves time and, if done right, saves money. There are several off-price catalogs to choose from. Think about it: no searching for a parking space. No public dressing rooms. All you need is just a quiet place to sit and thumb through the latest entry in your mailbox. Lots of mainstream retailers put out catalogs. Check to see if your favorite stores have a catalog. If so, get on the list.

STOP 3: INTERNET. You can shop from the convenience of your home 24/7 for practically anything on the World Wide Web. Think of shopping on the Internet like catalog shopping, without having to turn a page! Again, many of the mainstream retailers have Web sites. Some sites have virtual models where you can put in your measurements and the site will show you how the garment will look on you. An as an added bonus, often they have special sales exclusively for their e-mail customers. There are tons of beauty and fashion online newsletters that you can subscribe to. There are lots of advantages to being a subscriber. You will know about the sales at the different companies before the general public does; the site may offer special savings exclusively to its readership; and other companies may tandem up to offer special deals as well.

STEP 4: TELEVISION HOME SHOPPING. What a great way to shop in your robe while you are doing your pedicure. There are several home shopping channels to choose from. The quality has greatly increased over the years, as lots of designers have realized that this is a great medium in which to present their latest season offerings. And since the channels buy the garments in bulk, the clothing can be offered at much less cost that you can get—for the same item—in the retail store.

STOP 5: EBAY. This is the queen of auction sites. You can shop until you drop—or at least until your mouse finger can no longer click. The sky is the limit on what you will find—designer goods, estate sales—you name it, and somebody will sell it. You can enter your size, what you are looking for, and even if you want only new items with tags. There are some cautions, so be careful. You might think that you are the highest bidder, when suddenly, in the last few seconds, someone outbids you. Also, most of the merchandise is not returnable. It is best to buy from eBay sellers with lots of good feedback, which is listed on the site.

STOP 6: DEPARTMENT STORE OUTLETS. Don't think of this as a place where clothing that did not sell goes to die a slow death. Sometimes it's just that it didn't move fast enough, or it had to be removed to allow new merchandise to be stocked. There are even malls in which every store is an outlet for some "mother ship" stores. Talk about a CZ dream!

STOP 7: BASEMENT/CLEARANCE STORES. Name-brand merchandise can be found at discounted prices. You may need to do a little searching, but with patience the find is often worth the wait. It is important to note that you need to really look at alterations. A missing button can drastically reduce the price tag, but you need to factor in the cost of replacing the missing button, or of alterations.

STOP 8: FACTORY OUTLET STORES. There are more than 350 factory outlets across the country. Clothing factories send merchandise to their outlets for the same reasons a retail store would. Overstock and/or new merchandise needs to be stocked. You can find many a good bargain on designer clothing, but beware, as some outlet manufacturers make goods just for their outlet stores, so you might not be getting true retail-level designer goods. Careful sleuthing is needed to determine if the item is the real deal. When in doubt, don't buy. There will be lots of other bargains down the pike.

STOP 9: OFF-PRICE SHOPPING. There are lots and lots of stores to choose from—practically one in every strip shopping mall around. Off-price stores are the perfect place to pick up brand-new, quality goods for less. These stores purchase end-of-the-season fashions from department and specialty stores, as well as overruns from manufacturers. This allows you to save a lot while you shop a lot.

STOP 10: BIG BOX STORES. You can "Target" the ones that come to mind. With their big-buck budgets, these big box stores can offer lots of fashion for very little bucks. Make it a habit to walk the isles to see what is new and what is hot.

STOP 11: THRIFT STORES. Like consignment stores, thrift stores offer a treasure chest of dressing diamonds—if you have the time. Find a thrift store in a neighborhood that is young and hip. That is the best way to "find the find" you are looking for.

STOP 12: FRIENDLY EXCHANGE. Why not have a clothes-swapping party? What a great time to bring friends and great clothing together! You could serve fresh fruit and a little wine while you "shop" one another's wardrobes. It is so much fun to try on different outfits. And think about the guilt that will be saved from throwing out clothes when instead you can let another person enjoy them. In this case, the old saying "Your trash can be someone else's treasures" holds true.

STOP 13: YOUR VERY OWN CLOSET. How about updating a garment from your own closet? If the sleeves are too short on a jacket, cut them off, and you can literally create a vest suit in no time. If you are crafty, crocheting and knitting is hot, especially in vest and sweaters. Another terrific idea is to create a no-sew blouse for a suit. Buy one yard of beautiful material with the color of your suit in it. Simply drape it around your neck. Crisscross it on your bust and pin it to your undergarments. The effect is very chic and sophisticated, without the extra bulk of a blouse underneath. But you must remember—even if your jacket catches fire—do not remove it!

DRESSING DIAMONDS

No matter what your fashion personality, classic dressing is timeless. It is synonymous with simple and chic and is never, ever, boring. Think Audrey Hepburn, Catherine Deneuve, Jackie O—all were always impeccably dressed. Even when wearing the latest styles, all of these fashion icons were classics.

Once you have a few classic pieces in your closet, you can throw them on at a moment's notice, or build an entire outfit around them, using your wardrobe basics. Classics and basics are the core of what elegant—and effortless—dressing is all about.

The Basics

Clothing that is your wardrobe staple is considered a basic. It is the canvas on which you build your outfit. To build a basic wardrobe, start by choosing one color that really works for you. Navy, black, blue, green, or brown are good basic builders. Add two or three complementary colors such as beige, white, cream, and perhaps a metallic such as silver, bronze, or gold. This will form the combination on which you build. Basic items include:

- Blouses and tops. Choose ones in the complementary and basic wardrobe colors.
- T-shirts. Solid colors are the most versatile.
- Sweaters. Design elements can be pullover, turtlenecks, cardigans, etc.

- Slacks. Choose a couple of different styles such as tailored, dressy, and capri.
- Skirts. Best basics are knee length, and a longer one for style.

The Classics

These pieces are the featured stars of glamour dressing—your fashion statement pieces.

- **A three-piece suit.** Jacket, pants, and skirt in a solid color and all-season fabric.
- **Navy or red blazer.** This item will make a statement every time you wear it.
- **White shirt.** A couple of crisp white shirts with design details like French cuffs and/or mandarin collars.
- **Khaki slacks.** Timeless and extremely wearable. A great alternative to jeans.
- **Jeans.** Every Glamour Girl needs a couple of pairs of classic jeans. To keep them classic, keep them pressed.
- **Cashmere sweaters.** These items never go out of style and they always look like the latest in fashion, making their price well worth it. Invest in one or two. You'll wear them so often, and for so long, they will definitely prove to be worth their cost.
- **Twin sets.** Solid-color twin sweater sets are wonderful to mix it up.
- **Little black dress.** Where would fashion be without the LBD?

The great thing about having a basic and classic wardrobe is that you will always look stylish and—most important—you will always have something to wear!

ACCENT ON ACCESSORIES

The secrets of style lie in choosing clothes and producing outfits that express your style and personality. Details make the difference. A classic little black dress can create many different looks simply by changing accessories. An understated strand of pearls creates the allure of the country club scene. That same dress adorned with a colorful splashy scarf tied at the waist gives an artsy, carefree feel. And for the evening out, you can add the Midas touch by lavishing on layers of gold and glitz.

When you choose accessories, it is important to remember the scale and size of the items in relation to your body size. For example, if you are tall or full figured, your accessories should be larger than those for someone of petite stature. The look needs to be balanced so as not to overpower or underpower an outfit.

Fashion experts agree that the best dressers spend two-thirds of their clothing dollars on accessories and only one-third on clothing, and it's true. Think about the little black dress example. Just by changing the accessories, you can create at least three different looks. Accessories fall into seven categories:

1. **Shoes.** You will need three pairs: black, neutral, and a colorful flat. The best investment a glamour girl can make is a classic pump shoe. It fits each and every occasion. Real leather is a must. It wears well, is much more comfortable, and will long outlast shoes made of synthetics.

2. **Handbags.** You will need a black and a neutral bag, and leather, once again, is a must. Style and shape need to be in proportion to your body. Don't overstuff your handbag. It should not be your portable filing cabinet. It breaks the proportional lines and looks stuffy and cluttered.

3. **Belts.** Own at least two. A classic black leather and a gold or silver chain will add versatility to many outfits.

4. **Earrings.** Metallic and pearl earrings are a wardrobe staple. However, colorful earrings are one of the most inexpensive ways to bring color to your outfits.

5. **Necklaces.** A strand of pearls—real or costume—is a must. Add some gold and colored stone ones for accent pieces.

6. **Pins.** Perfect for adding flair to an outfit. Mix your jewelry box with both classic and whimsical pieces. A pin is a calling card—people will comment.

7. **Scarves.** The most colorful and inexpensive way to change an outfit, scarves can be tied at the neck, around the waist, or draped dramatically over the shoulders. The looks you can create with a scarf are endless. And remember, take them out of the drawers and put them in your closet. Believe it or not, a plastic six-pack holder makes an excellent scarf rack. You simple drape several scarves through the openings and place them on a hanger. When you see them, you will wear them.

Think about the last time you bragged to a friend about the cost of an outfit. It is safe to venture that it was about how much you saved or the great price you paid. There isn't a woman alive who doesn't love a bargain—whether her banking account contains lots of commas or just a decimal point! But as Thrifty Girls, we knew that all along. And finally, I present to you The Rules.

To get the most for your shopping dollar follow The Rules:

1. Do not buy anything—ever—that doesn't make you look and feel your very best.

2. If you would not pay full price for it, don't buy it on sale.

3. If you have to think about it or talk yourself into it, let it go.

4. Always try it on and view yourself in a three-way mirror. And for goodness' sake, sit down in it in front of the mirror to see what others see.

5. If you do not have one single thing that it will go with— put it back. You do not need any one-hit wonders.

6. Never shop under pressure. Allow plenty of time to find the outfit for the big event.

Armed with these rules, you should always be able to stay true to your Thrifty Girl self, while looking like a total Glamour Girl.

Chapter Twenty-six

Thirty Thrifty Tips to Dressing Svelte

" She looked as if she had been poured into her clothes and had forgotten to say 'when.' "

—P. G. WODEHOUSE

I f you are built like a movie star or model, or have the dimensions somewhere along the lines of 36-24-36, I am sorry to say it, but you will have to leave. This information is highly confidential and only for those of us in the 99 percent of the world who aren't built like models.

How come movie stars are the only ones who get to pick and choose the images they portray? Movie stars get to sign off on a picture before it is released. We, on the other hand, cannot edit out our figure flaws. Here are thirty dressing svelte tips that are sure to make your entrance a grand one!

1. Stand up straight. This automatically squares off your shoulders, pulls in your tummy, and lengthens the line of your body. You will look pounds lighter instantly.

2. Get a full-length mirror. Check yourself out, front and back, in the full-length mirror. Often it's the rear view—a skirt that cups your bottom, a pleat that won't lie flat—that advertises pounds, and somehow you are the only one who does not notice.

3. Say it with me: Wear darker colors. Dark colors are the ultimate slimmer.

4. Buy a great bra. Look for a bra that keeps the fullest part of your bosom exactly halfway between shoulder and waist—check your profile in the mirror. When your bust line falls lower, you get a short-waisted, matronly effect and clothes do not fit properly.

5. When you want to, wear light. Light or bright colors, when worn monochromatically, give the longest, leanest line.

6. Match your hosiery. In order to elongate your silhouette even more, wear hosiery that matches your hemline and shoe color. (But common sense is needed—no bright red, purple, or stark-white pantyhose—EVER!) Choose a sheer taupe to shadow and slim the legs if matching is out of the question.

7. Be well-heeled. Whenever appropriate, wear heels to add a few slenderizing inches of height.

8. Skim the body. Buy clothes that skim the body comfortably and are no bigger or wider than they have to be. It just isn't true that tight clothes will make you seem smaller (or that you will diet your way into them). And you cannot hide out in humongous clothes—you will just look humongous.

9. Rethink your hair. If it is very long, full, or fussy, it may be accenting your size instead of drawing attention away from it. Stand in front of a full-length mirror—at least 5 feet away—and study its effect on your silhouette. A shorter, simpler cut with a little height on top might make your neck (and you) seem longer and slimmer.

10. Don't add unnecessary bulk. Think seriously about thick tweeds, fluffy knit or stiff fabrics. Look instead for flat knits and material that drape in an easy, fluid way without clinging.

11. Avoid dropped-shoulder styles. They create a horizontal line that widen and shorten the upper body, add pounds, and rule out the magic of shoulder pads.

12. Wear thin shoulder pads. Whenever possible, pop some in. Pads make clothes drape better, help hide any little budges around bra straps in back, and create a visual balance that minimizes hips and waist.

13. If your waist is proportionally tiny. . . . Please avoid the temptation to show it off with bright or tight belts; they could make everything above and below look bigger.

14. The longer your skirt . . . Remember the long and short of it. The shorter your jacket, the longer your skirt, or vice versa.

15. Stick with long sleeves. Long sleeves are always more slimming than short ones.

16. Pantsuits create height. Pantsuits make everyone look taller and slimmer. This is especially important to remember if you are petite.

17. Avoid excess details. Generally, things like ruffles, gathers, pleats, piping, and patch pockets add pounds.

18. Think twice. Before you tuck, think—is this making me look thinner? When in doubt, leave it out.

19. Control-top pantyhose. Gifts from the slimming fairy, control-top pantyhose really work. And if you haven't tried them under slacks, you should. They give a slimmer, smoother line in seconds.

20. Footless control-top pantyhose. The newest sweet slimmer is footless control-top pantyhose that allow you to be able to wear your sandals without worry. They cover from the waist to where you want them to end—ankle or calf; it's your choice, as you can put them where you want them to end.

21. Accessory necessary. Choose jewelry, handbags, and shoes that are in proportion to your body; very small, delicate accessories make large women look larger. (But don't let a bulky shoulder bag hang at your hips if they are your widest point. Shorten the strap or switch to a handheld bag.)

22. Avoid chokers. Chokers create an unflattering horizontal line. Long chains and ropes of pearls or beads will look much better.

23. Go for the angles. Large rounded pins and earrings call attention to rounded proportions; geometric shapes and off-center placement are more slimming.

24. A simple, narrow belt. Simple and narrow is the slim ticket. Choose one that matches your dress, skirt, or pants for the most slenderizing choice. If you want to show off a belt with a beautiful buckle, wear it under an open jacket or cardigan to define your waist without giving away the whole story.

25. Always bend way over. Exercise your way to a great fit. Bend over and sit down in any new garment before buying it. Clothes should not ride up in the back or pull tightly across the shoulders, chest, or hips.

26. Under cover. A large bulky label can create an unwelcome bulge behind the neckline. Simply cut it out.

27. Create the element of disguises. Choose a swimsuit that provides a needed distraction. For example, if your hips are a "problem" area, find a suit with a fashion element at the top.

28. Talk it up. Talk with experienced salespeople. Wardrobe consultants are often available in shops and department stores. They can be a valuable resource when analyzing your own figure strengths and flaws.

29. Chuck the chunky. Do not wear platform shoes! In fact, avoid all chunky footwear altogether. Simple, low-cut classic pumps help legs look longer.

30. Take a deep breath. Try to buy natural fabrics that breathe, such as cotton or linen, rather than polyester. Being comfortable in your clothing, especially in hot weather, is a must.

INDEX

flyaway hair, 42
foot care, 156–61, 174, 176
footwear, 217, 222, 224
fougeres, 140–41
foundation, 83–86, 113
fragrance, 138–46, 176
fungal infections, 158

G

gel blush, 90
green tea, 76

H

hair accessories, 43
hair color
    bargains, 3–4
    choosing, 7
    at home, 4–11
    maintenance tips, 9–10
    types of, 5–6
hair extensions, 24
hair masks, 39
hair part, 13, 40
hair removal, 132–34
hair salons, finding specials at,
    27–28
hairstyles
    bobs, 20, 41
    facial shape and, 13–20
    hiding flaws, 22–23
    importance of right, 32–33
    length, 34–35
    lifestyle and, 20–22
    maintaining, 33–34
hairstylists
    communicating with, 29–
    30, 32, 35–37

finding right, 24, 26–28
hair tips, 38–43
handbags, 217
hand care, 148–54, 175–76
hand washing, 174
hats, 40, 41
healthy lifestyle, 79
heart faces, 15–16
height
    accentuating, 187–88
    deaccentuating, 188
highlights, 6, 9
hips, 190
hosiery, 221–22, 223
hourglass body shape, 186–87

I

Internet shopping, 212
inverted heart faces, 19–20

J

jewelry, 218, 223–24

L

laser whitening treatments, 168
lash thickeners, 119
layered cuts, 34
layering, 35
legs, 190–91
lines, 56
lip brushes, 118
lip liners, 106–7, 115
lip lines, 56
lips, 76, 103–10
    makeup for, 103–8, 110–11,
    113, 117
    shapes of, 108–10

About Susie

Armed with quick wit, years of professional experience, and more get-pretty tips than a beauty pageant coordinator, Susie Galvez is an internationally known beauty expert and a leading consultant in the spa industry. The founder of a day spa in Richmond, Virginia, Susie is an esthetician, makeup artist, and the author of seven books on beauty, weight loss, and successful spa management.

She is a frequent speaker at international spa conventions and has been featured on radio and TV programs around the nation, as well as in publications such as *Allure, Elle, Good Housekeeping, Fitness, Self, Oxygen, Woman's World, Health, First for Women, Woman's Own,* and iVillage.com.

Inspired by the thrill she gets from helping women rediscover beauty on a daily basis, Susie is dedicated to giving women tools to help them accept themselves and realize that each day is another chance to be beautiful. To learn more about Susie, log onto *www.susiegalvez.com.*

In between writing and speaking, Susie is hard at work with Hello Beautiful, (*www.hellobeautifulspa.com*) her national skincare line specializing in professional spa strength products designed at-home use. She and her spa have been featured in trade publications such as *Dermascope, Les Nouvelle Esthetique, Salon Today, American Spa, Modern Salon, Skin, Inc., Nails, Nails Plus,* and *Day Spa magazine.*

And if all that isn't enough to keep Susie constantly on the go, she is also and active member of Cosmetic Executive Women, the National Association of Women Business Owners, and the Society of American Cosmetic Chemists.